Power
Pranayama

Second
Edition
with exclusive
video links
inside

Power Pranayama

DISCOVER THE HEALING POTENTIAL OF YOUR BREATH

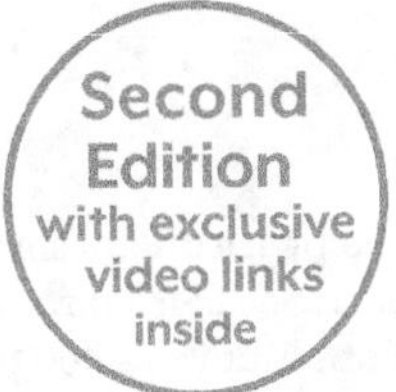

DR RENU MAHTANI
WITH MEETA KABRA

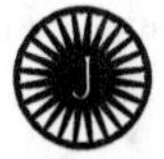

JAICO PUBLISHING HOUSE

Ahmedabad Bangalore Chennai
Delhi Hyderabad Kolkata Mumbai

Published by Jaico Publishing House
A-2 Jash Chambers, 7-A Sir Phirozshah Mehta Road
Fort, Mumbai - 400 001
jaicopub@jaicobooks.com
www.jaicobooks.com

POWER PRANAYAMA
ISBN 978-93-93559-56-2

First Jaico Impression: 2023

Page design and layout by R. Ajith Kumar, Delhi

CONTENTS

Contents

HOW DO WE GET THERE

AUTHOR'S NOTE

Through this book, we hope to convey what we have learnt so far about how our breath affects our well-being. Our knowledge about breath from Indian scriptures and modern medicine are a beacon guiding us towards the best health possible.

With that in mind, the first section looks at our state of health, given our lifestyle and stressors. Most of us know that we have health concerns that need to be addressed but don't know where to start. We have the solution, literally, at the tip of our nose, in the form of our breath. This is where we are right now.

Then, we discuss the knowledge available to us in the form of existing wisdom in ancestral texts and modern medicine—both of which are vast beyond measure. We will briefly introduce the know-how and mesmerising interconnections of the various parts of the body. From our study of modern medicine, it is indeed beautiful to realise why our ancestors experiments worked. This is where we want to be: a stage where our body functions as intended, given our limitations.

The last section mentions practices you can easily incorporate into your lifestyle. It includes preparing the body through correct posture and breathing, and then use specific breathing techniques over 15–20 minutes everyday that will guide you to good health.

WHERE WE ARE NOW

ONE

OUR LIFESTYLE, STRESS AND ILLNESS

Good health is what nature intended for us.

As a student of modern medicine, I was taught a lot about disease. I wish I was also taught about good health. As a practitioner, I now know that specialisations are necessary, but there is a gaping hole in understanding holistic health. As a patient of modern lifestyle diseases, I know that to a large extent, I can be in control of my own health. Being in good health should be the norm. Any deviation from good health needs healing. Nature itself provides our body with biological processes to heal. Re-joining of fractured bones, recovery from a fever, coagulation of blood, are all examples of such healing.

Medicines consumed at this time serve two purposes: they alleviate pain, or they prevent or treat secondary infections.

When the healing process falters or leaves scars behind, your mental faculties help you accept the situation. From being diagnosed with a fatal disease to dealing with a close one's death, our mental health determines how we cope.

As it stands, not too many people can claim that they are in good health. Nature bestows some health issues upon us while others are due to external factors like accidents, etc. We open ourselves to yet other illnesses with our lifestyles and the accompanying stress. The last set of diseases are preventable to a large extent.

However, we need to think of health beyond mere absence of disease. Good health is the optimal state of bodily functions. It is also the body's ability to respond correctly to an ever-changing environment. Our lungs, heart, liver and other organs are all designed to deal with frequent changes. Good health allows these organs to continue to function well despite these changes by adapting to them.

What then, keeps these organs from functioning optimally? Common ailments are classified according to the bodily system that failed.

Degenerative diseases such as diabetes, multiple sclerosis, and muscular degeneration result from our organs losing the capacity to function the way they are supposed to. Auto-immune disorders include thyroid-related issues, various skin diseases, and rheumatism, among many others. In such ailments, our immune system gets confused enough to start attacking our own body. Allergies are both a cause and effect of a weakened immune system. New infections constantly surface and show greater resistance to the widening array of antibiotics.

Lifestyle-related ailments such as hypertension, peptic ulcers, colitis, and IBS (Irritable Bowel Syndrome) arise and stay throughout our lives. Increasingly, young people have begun to suffer from heart disease. Over-eating and an unhealthy diet leading to obesity has become commonplace.

Irrespective of how they are classified, the root cause for these diseases is untraceable. There are always multiple factors and no definitive culprit. This could be partially tracked back to the all-encompassing source: stress.

While healthy habits in terms of fitness and diet are becoming a part of our routines, we remain aware that we can fall prey to any of the above diseases at any time. We then look towards modern medicine and other 'pathies' to provide a cure. Unfortunately, I have realised that many of these treatments are incomplete.

However, a holistic approach to health has the potential to lead us to an answer. Under this approach, it is believed that diseases and ailments originate deep within the body before they appear physically and mentally. This happens because of an imbalance in one bodily system or the other.

That said, the human mind's capacity to participate in the body's healing process is what we wish to tap through the techniques presented in this book.

Before we get a basic understanding of bodily systems, both modern and ancient, let us understand why many a disease has "stress" as either a cause or an effect.

STRESS AND ILLNESS

Let's break the illness-stress-illness cycle.

Even if we assume that the first sign of an ailment had no particular root cause, no one can deny that the condition will cause stress. Stress by itself—if it presents itself in mild forms or infrequently—isn't a threat. The human body has evolved to cope with some amount of stress. Unfortunately, most of us experience intense stress. All. The. Time.

Let us take a look at why this happens. Human beings respond to the outside world in such a way that every input to our senses triggers a part of the brain. The brain, in turn, instructs the body's organs to take action. So, the sight and smell of an ice cream cone or a burger trigger sensory nerves from the eyes and the nose to the brain with information on the food item. Our brain then instructs the salivary glands in the mouth to produce more saliva. A similar connection of reflex nerves makes us pull our hands back with an immediate jerk when we touch something hot. These instantaneous responses of the body to harmful threats form the basis of our survival instinct. They are important.

In primitive times, for survival in the jungle, our brain was attuned to meet external challenges like wild animals by triggering a fight-or-flight response in the body. This would enable the body to recruit physiological changes to cope with the demand of either fighting the threat or fleeing from it.

Clearly, stress is unavoidable. In fact, short-term, manageable stress is good for us as it helps build our coping mechanism like planning our day, having and nurturing a baby, a new job or an exciting project. We can develop skills and gain confidence to handle challenges over time to manage such stress. This good stress helps us grow and feel our best. Short-term stress can even boost the health of cells, a phenomenon called hormesis or toughening. Such beneficial stress is known as 'eustress'.

The ups and downs of daily life usually do not wear the body out, unless we are hypersensitive or over-reactive by nature. However, if the stress is intense or becomes chronic, it can take a toll. Such stress can result from job burnout, prolonged anger and resentment, financial crisis, the death of a loved one, health concerns, bad relationships, etc. These negative stressors commonly called 'distress' are the genesis for many ailments.

If we move from one stress to another: from the lane-cutter on the road to the existence of traffic which we are ourselves a part of; the bickering boss to family pressure; the struggle between "Netflix" and the "fear of missing out"—our stress becomes chronic and adds up to become much more intense than any single event causing stress.

We offer our body some high quality stress. And lots of it.

Our body is not meant to constantly deal with such stress.

Most of these stressors make fighting or fleeing socially inappropriate. What do we do then, in the face of such modern stressors? We fight with words or we freeze! Often, we suppress the physical reaction to the stressor to override it or we over-react and burn ourselves out.

Since we are constantly dealing with one distress event or another, the physiological changes used by the body to cope are always in "on" mode. They don't get a chance to rest. The all-important stress-response is thus over-used. Our organs and systems are not meant to handle perpetual stress—neither in terms of quality nor quantity. Therefore, the system starts giving way to aches and pains, diseases and ailments.

This starts a stress-illness-stress-illness cycle that needs to break.

And break it, we can.

We are a unique set of generations with two powerful sets of knowledge at our disposal. We know more about how our body functions than we ever have, thanks to modern medicine. At the same time, our ancestors have left behind a treasure trove with practical techniques and philosophical wisdom that we can use to cope with our physical and mental health issues.

WHERE WE WANT TO BE

KNOWLEDGE FROM MODERN MEDICINE

Our journey to being in and maintaining good health begins with understanding how systems in the body work, individually and together. Modern medicine has taken huge strides in the last couple of centuries and continues to discover layers of details at an even faster pace. From diagnostics to investigation and early detection of diseases, modern medicine has controlled the spread and treated many a life-threatening infectious disease. Technological advancements like laparoscopic surgery have led to fewer complications and failure rates. All these advances have considerably increased the average lifespan.

We have also discovered that there are physiological mechanisms in our body through which chronic stress and associated emotional states contribute to physical diseases. Of the various systems that come together to make our body what it is, the nervous system, the endocrine system, and the respiratory system are particularly relevant to our understanding of pranayama, as discussed later in the book.

Each cell of the body receives input from these three systems in the form of nerve stimulus, hormones and oxygen, respectively. The nervous system is responsible for receiving and sending signals to various organs of the body. The endocrine system produces hormones, which in turn try to balance other chemicals in the body. The organs of the respiratory system move oxygen through the body into the cells and expel carbon dioxide out of the body.

We will now take a better look at these systems. However, do remember that this is a very brief bird's eye view and far from being comprehensive. The descriptions below give you an overall understanding of the systems involved when you practice pranayama.

NERVOUS SYSTEM → NERVES

We aren't really a ball of nerves.
At least, we are not meant to be.

ANATOMY AND PHYSIOLOGY

CENTRAL NERVOUS SYSTEM: THE MAIN SUPPLY LINE

Think of our brain as a supercomputer that initiates action, processes the result and causes more action. Thus the brain's activities are both cause and effect of its interaction with the outer world.

From the brain originates a major cable, our spinal cord, that runs down to the end of our torso, the trunk of our body. The brain and the spinal cord make one part of the nervous system, the **central nervous system (CNS)**. The CNS controls the activities of the body through neurons starting from the brain and reaching every nook and corner of the physical body. Normal functioning of the nervous system results in good physical health enabling the body and all its organs to carry out the decisions of the mind. You would recall the manner in which human beings interact with the world.

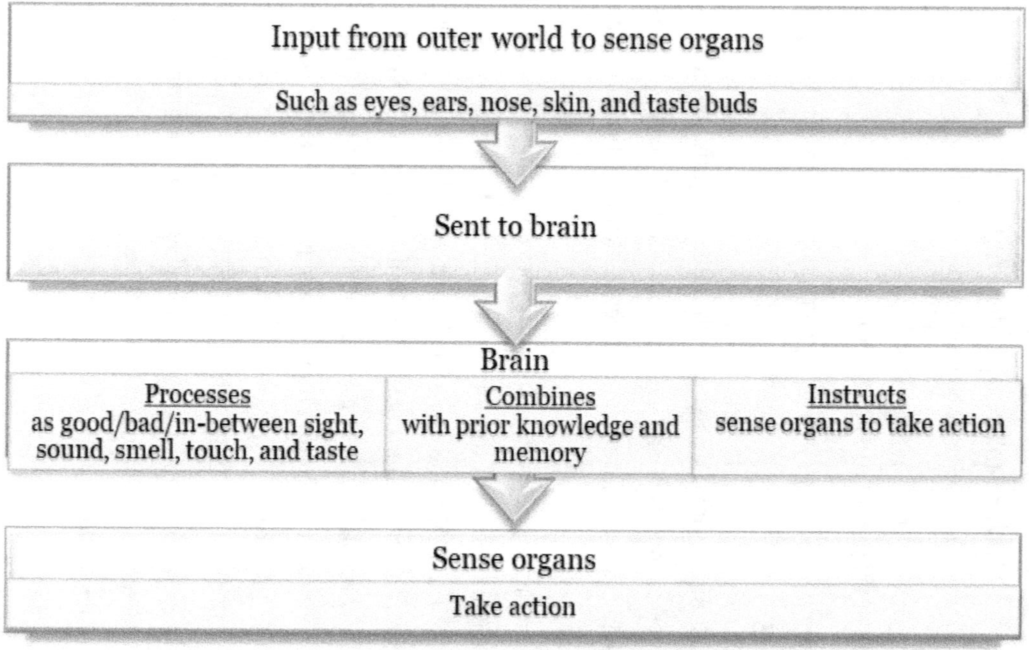

The brain's interaction with the outer world

Similarly, the stress response affects the body through the nervous system too. The anxious discontented mind, exhausts and irritates the nervous system and the body fails to function efficiently when the mind is in a state of stress. In this way, mental stress produces disease and degeneration.

HYPOTHALAMUS: THE BEHIND-THE-SCENE MANAGER

The hypothalamus is a part deeply buried in the brain, close to its centre. Information is transmitted to the hypothalamus from every body part, including the sense centres in the brain itself. It analyses the information received, decides the response and the changes needed in the body, and instructs the relevant cells to carry out the decisions it has made.

The hypothalamus can be considered as the director of not only the nervous system, but also the hormonal system because it produces the "controlling" hormones. These hormones not only regulate body processes such as metabolism, but they also control the release of hormones from other endocrine glands like the thyroid, the adrenals and the sex glands.

Among many other functions, the hypothalamus maintains a stable body temperature, controls blood pressure, ensures fluid balance and even a good sleeping pattern. The expression of emotions such as fear and anger is partly controlled by the hypothalamus.

The hypothalamus is a unique bridge between the nervous system and the endocrine system. We will discuss this later.

PERIPHERAL NERVOUS SYSTEM: THE REACH PROGRAMME

The other part of the nervous system is a network of nerves sprouting out of the spinal cord, linking the brain to every part of the body. This is called the **peripheral nervous system**.

A simple example of how these two sub-systems work in tandem is when you see food that you like. The nerves in the eyes send a pulse to the brain with information on the visual. The brain processes this and relays back an impulse to the glands in your mouth, instructing them to produce saliva. Such relaying of information and decision-making happens for every little action your body takes. It happens when you look at clothes in a shop and your brain decides to buy them or not, when you hear a voice you don't like and you feel annoyed, and so on.

Broadly, every organ functions in a similar fashion. Your brain sends signals to your respiratory system to breathe, to your digestive system to take in food and pass on what it doesn't need to the excretory system, and so on.

As you might have noticed, you can control some of these responses voluntarily while others happen automatically. The peripheral nervous system operates through two different sub-systems to take care of the voluntary and involuntary functions, respectively—the somatic nervous system and the autonomic nervous system (ANS).

SOMATIC NERVOUS SYSTEM: THINGS WE CONTROL

The somatic nervous system controls voluntary muscles and transmits sensory information to the CNS. This is the part of the nervous system that commands the reflex action when you touch something hot. This part of the nervous system is also responsible for sensory actions such as sight, hearing, smelling, taste and touch. Other examples of voluntary activities, that is, actions you can control include walking, writing, and turning your neck from side to side.

AUTONOMIC NERVOUS SYSTEM: THE ELVES AT WORK

This controls involuntary functions of the body, that is, functions that you cannot control. For instance, digestion, sweating, pumping of the heart, happen on their own, controlled by the ANS.

Many of the organs involved, such as the stomach, sweat glands, heart, etc. are required to do two things depending on the external environment. They either allow the body to fight or fly away from a given situation, as would happen if you see an insect that you don't like. Or they need the body to relax and rest when the external environment is free of threats. Accordingly, the ANS is further categorised into two wings.

Sympathetic Nervous System (SNS): Fight or Flight

This system gives the body signals to either fight or run away from a threat in the environment. It plays a dominant role when you experience stress by altering the heart rate, blood pressure, oxygen consumption, respiration, constrict blood vessels, pupillary dilation, sweating, etc. to prepare the body for the fight or flight response. The brain does the needful automatically, and you usually don't have much control. Keep in mind the word "usually".

Parasympathetic Nervous System (PNS): Rest and Relax

Your body needs to rest and relax too. This part of the autonomic nervous system automatically soothes and restores normalcy to all bodily functions by conserving and restoring energy. This leads to a normalisation of the increased heart rate, blood pressure, pupil dilation, etc. The body now has the energy to allow functions that were on hold under stress, such as digestive processes and the elimination of bodily waste.

Most of the organs inside the body are supplied by the nerves from both sets of the ANS nerves. After the somatic nervous system has dealt with the threat, the PNS takes over to revert the body to its original state. This prepares you to deal with the next threat when the somatic nervous system takes over organ functioning again. And so goes the circle. By countering the effects of each other, the two wings of the ANS establish a balanced state called homeostasis.

HOMEOSTASIS, HARMONY, AND OUR INTERFERENCE

This is an opportune moment to recall the thought we left the last chapter with. We offer our body some high-quality stress. And lots of it. Our body is not meant to deal with constant stress.

The body's systems are supposed to get stressed when the body is stimulated. When faced with a threat, your SNS is meant to trigger a rise in the heart rate, the sugar level in the blood, and blood pressure so that the body has the energy to deal with the threat. Similarly, the pupils need to dilate to see better, the breath rate should increase to take in more oxygen, and so on.

But once the threat has passed, the systems have to be given time to recuperate. The PNS has to bring back to normalcy all the stimulated functions mentioned above.

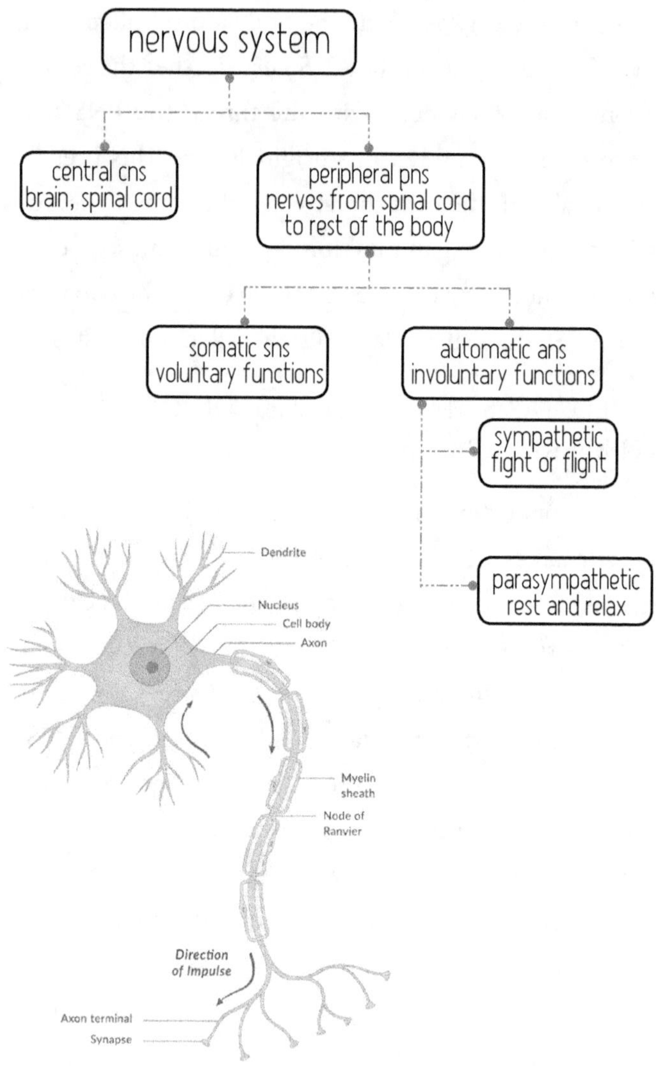

The Nervous System

Ideally, everything goes back to an in-between state, a state of homeostasis, a state of harmony.

Unfortunately, our habits have evolved to keep the body in a constantly triggered or stimulated stress state. That means that our body faces the stress from our job but doesn't get a break before it faces the stress at home because there is road rage on the way. As a result, functions such as blood pressure, heart rate, and sugar levels are constantly stimulated. They do not have the time to recover.

The good news is that not all functions collapse. The bad news is each of us has a relatively weaker function that cannot hold up to the stress any longer. This weakness might be due to genetics or just our natural disposal. Irrespective of the reason, the weak function stops working the way it is supposed to. So, if we have a family or personal history of blood pressure staying up, that gives way, and we suffer from high blood pressure. The same goes for blood sugar, acidity, etc.

Over time, this imbalance leads to an imbalance in other systems too, as they are all interconnected. One of these is the endocrine system.

ENDOCRINE SYSTEM → HORMONES

Yes, it is all hormonal.

In our body are groups of cells called glands that produce chemicals and substances called hormones. For example, sweat glands produce a substance called sweat, and mammary glands produce milk for new-borns. Similarly, the salivary glands produce saliva, and the prostate glands produce semen.

The various substances above are produced and exit the body. Another set of glands produce substances called hormones, which are used within the body itself. This group of glands that produces hormones is called the endocrine system.

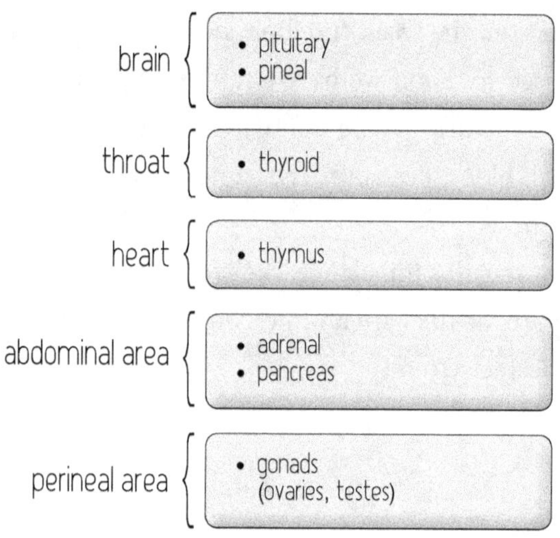

Parts of the endocrine system

Hormones travel through the blood and facilitate many bodily functions such as metabolism, growth, and sexual development.

While the list above is not an exhaustive one by far, these are some of the major endocrine glands. Do note the location of these glands. Especially as it relates to the discussion so far, the pituitary gland is located inside the hypothalamus area of the brain.

This is why the hypothalamus is the unique bridge between the nervous system and the endocrine system. It provides stimulus to both systems. The systems, in turn, stimulate nerves and produce hormones, which all supply input to each cell of the body to perform their functions.

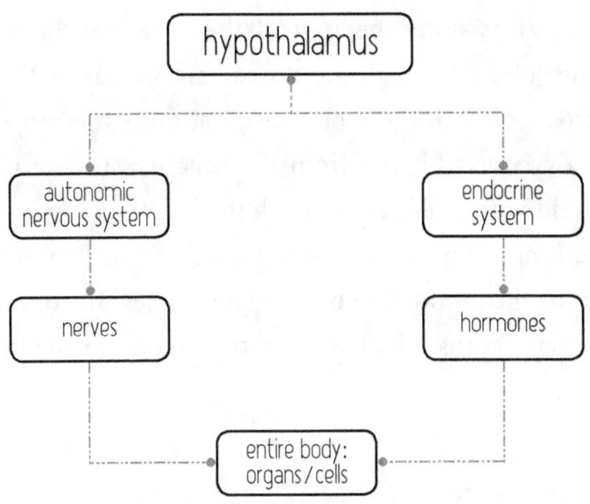

The unique bridge between the nervous system and the endocrine system

Again, the disharmony caused by our constantly stressed lifestyles is responsible for the all-too-familiar hormonal imbalance. The reach and impact of hormones is so vast and deep that it has been difficult so far for modern science to identify direct cause and effect relationships between many illnesses and the hormonal imbalance that might cause them.

Yet, all is not lost. We have a tool at our disposal that can relieve us from our illnesses, if not minimise or eliminate them altogether. Our breath.

RESPIRATORY SYSTEM → BREATH

Our breath is the grand connector between our outer and inner worlds.

The respiratory system begins with the air we breathe in from the atmosphere through the nose. This air passes through the throat to reach the lungs. Respiration is the process in which oxygen is filtered from the breath you take in and carbon dioxide is filtered out with the breath you release.

The lungs employ an in-built mechanism to move the oxygen to the blood. The blood then carries this oxygen to the various organs, which enables them to perform multiple functions.

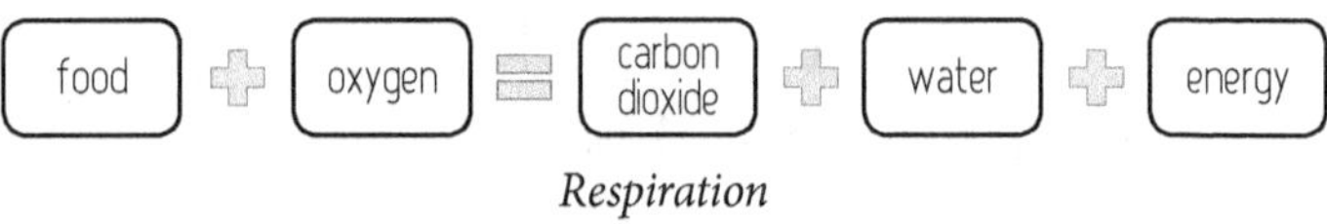

Respiration

THE MECHANICS OF BREATHING

Our body needs energy on a large scale for its day-to-day activities. Food is a vital source of energy, but this energy is not absorbed directly. To convert this energy into a functional form, oxygen is required. Without oxygen, energy cannot be extracted even from the best of foods. In the presence of oxygen, nutrients in food are burnt or broken down in our cells to liberate usable energy. The carbon dioxide produced in the process gets discarded subsequently.

The energy obtained is used to drive each and every function of the body. These functions are collectively called metabolic functions. Thus, all activities are performed with the help of the breath. One can live for two months without food and two weeks without water, but only a few minutes without air.

Breathing or respiration cyclically takes place in four steps: inhalation, pause, exhalation, pause. We inhale to absorb the oxygen that is needed to convert food into energy. When we exhale, we not only discard carbon dioxide and impurities but also create space for new air. This entire process of exchanging oxygen and carbon dioxide is controlled by nerves, which carry signals from the respiratory control areas of the brain.

Let us understand the respiration process and its intermingling with the body's other systems, including *prana*, in greater detail. This will still merely be the surface level understanding of how things work. However, it will give us enough information to understand our pranayama practice better.

MUSCLES OF RESPIRATION

An inhalation begins in our nose, passes through the throat and reaches our lungs. The exhalation backtracks this route to let the air out of our nose. The primary muscles for free-flowing breaths are the intercostal muscles, the diaphragm and the abdominal muscles. We will get to each of these in a bit.

Some neck, shoulder and upper back muscles also come into play during extreme activity; these are the secondary breathing muscles. Unfortunately, some of us use these secondary muscles more than the primary ones, leading to shoulder and upper back tension.

intercostal muscles

diaphragm

abdominal muscles

Muscles of Respiration

The **intercostal muscles** occupy the space between the ribs. They are connected to the spine at the back and the sternum (the breastbone) in the front. These muscles work in a group, lifting the ribs up and out during inhalation and letting them move inward and downward during passive exhalation. Healthy action of the intercostal muscles is vital for the health and flexibility of the spine. Inadequate movement of the ribs due to shallow breathing can cause the spine to become rigid and inflexible.

The **diaphragm** is a large dome-shaped, curtain-like muscle situated between the chest and the abdomen. The heart and the lungs lie above it, and the abdominal organs like the stomach and the liver lie directly underneath it. The diaphragm is attached to the lower end of the sternum, the six lower ribs, and through extensions to the upper lumbar vertebrae that make up the arch in the lower back. When the diaphragm moves freely, there is movement in all the structures to which it is attached, and the breath flows rhythmically.

The **abdominal muscles** not only support the abdominal organs and the lower back but also play an active part during exhalation. If we draw these muscles gently towards the spine, they give the diaphragm a little push so that it rises up and a large volume of impure air is expelled. Therefore, our abdominal muscles need to be strong and well-toned to do their work. Remember, however, that 'strong' does not mean rigid or tense. In fact, during normal inhalation, the muscles should be soft and relaxed so that the diaphragm's descent is not restricted.

None of the above muscles work by themselves. Their action is interdependent for every breath.

THE BREATHING PROCESS

During inhalation, the chest expands to take the new breath in. Simultaneously, the diaphragm is gently pushed into the abdominal space causing a partial vacuum in the chest area. As the diaphragm flattens its dome shape and descends into the abdomen, it displaces the abdominal organs beneath it to push the abdominal muscles in the belly area forward.

Therefore, an efficiently working diaphragm massages the liver, the stomach, the kidneys, the pancreas, the spleen, the gallbladder and the intestines. Its movement also massages the heart, which rests on top of the diaphragm, explaining how free, rhythmic and relaxed breathing helps maintain a healthy heart.

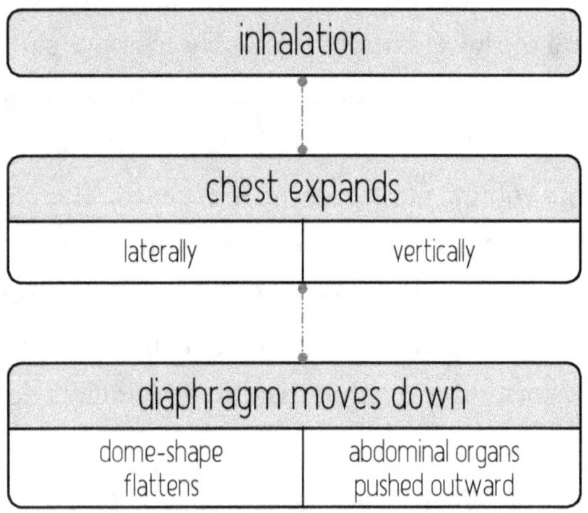

Muscular and organ movement with breath

CONTROLLING YOUR BREATH

Your nervous system is chiefly responsible for controlling and integrating a variety of bodily functions, including breathing. As you already know, normal spontaneous breathing takes place without us really being aware of it, without the intervention of our consciousness. So, even if you don't exert any control, it will keep doing its thing, and we will keep breathing.

But, as mentioned earlier, we can intervene in the process of breathing. And this power to intervene can be used for our physical well-being and peace of mind. We can deepen, hasten, smoothen our breaths with our conscious effort to do so. For instance, when we sing, we rapidly inhale through the mouth between strings of melody.

INVOLUNTARY CONTROL OF BREATHING

Our nervous system controls respiration by using a well-integrated hierarchy. The controls alter the rate and the depth of breathing to meet the varying oxygen demands of the body. This coordination is done with the help of a few 'centres' or specialised cells of the nervous system.

Without getting into too much technical detail, let us stick to their familiar names: the lower respiratory centre and the upper respiratory centre. The two centres are connected through the ANS.

LOWER RESPIRATORY CENTRE

The lower respiratory centre is situated in the lower part of the brain stem, where the skull unites with the neck. It maintains the breathing rhythm with the help of nerves passing through the spinal cord. These nerves connect to the muscles of breathing. Changes in the chemical composition of the blood directly affect the lower respiratory centre. Reduced oxygen, excess carbon dioxide, increased pH and acidity of the blood stimulate the centre to increase the rate and the depth of breathing, and vice versa.

You will also notice that, after jogging or any aerobic exercise, the breathing becomes faster and deeper. When you do cardio exercises, the body uses up oxygen much faster. Therefore, you need more oxygen. You also have to remove extra carbon dioxide produced as a result of increased metabolism in the exercising muscles.

UPPER RESPIRATORY CENTRE

This is where the hypothalamus is located. You might recall the importance of the hypothalamus. This tiny organ located deep between the two sides or hemispheres of the brain has rich nervous connections with various neuro-endocrine centres in the brain. The hypothalamus works through the autonomic nervous system to influence other centres, including the lower respiratory centre.

VOLUNTARY OR CONSCIOUS CONTROL OF BREATHING

The cortical control, the highest level of nerve control on breathing, comes from the frontal cortex of the brain. The frontal cortex is just behind the forehead and represents advancements in functions like higher emotions, perception, etc. As this specialised part of the brain has rich nerve connections with various parts of the brain, including the breathing centres, our breathing can be easily altered voluntarily or brought under conscious control. In other words, it can bring what is ordinarily instinctive into awareness or conscious control.

BREATH: BRINGING IT ALL TOGETHER

We can use the voluntary aspect of the nervous system to manipulate the breath, which in turn affects the involuntary functions conducted by the autonomic nervous system. That is, we can use our control on our breath to affect the functioning of our blood pressure, acidity, etc. Also, the breath influences the hypothalamus through the nervous system. And the hypothalamus, in turn, has access to the endocrine system. Therefore, the breath can be used to work on the production of hormones too.

So, you can manipulate your breath to calm down your heart rate when triggered by stress. This simple example can be extended to other lifestyle disorders too. Sure, each body, lifestyle, possible change, etc., is different, and no result can be guaranteed. All the same, it won't be far-fetched to say that breathing practices can manipulate involuntary responses to our advantage.

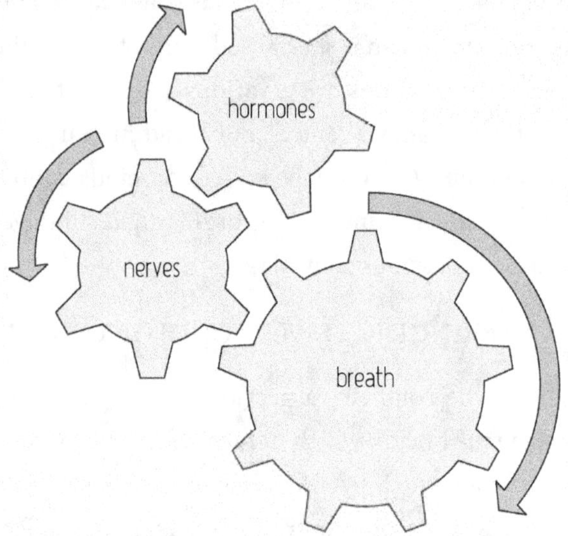

Breath: Bringing it all together

MEDICAL RESEARCH: A JOURNEY THAT DOESN'T END

**What we know is exciting.
What we don't know is mesmerising.**

What you've read so far, is just an extremely tiny glimpse of what we know about the body. And what we know is only a slim sliver of the many processes happening within the body. And no, the diagram below is not to scale.

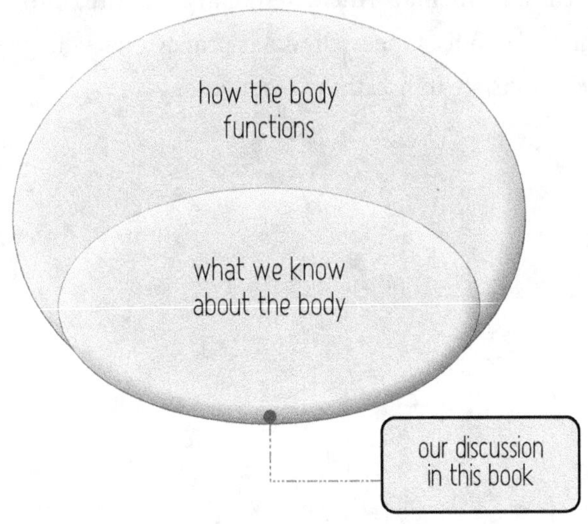

We know so little

Modern science too has a lot to discover, process, analyse and work out how the jigsaw puzzle fits—one with an infinite number of visible and invisible parts. Parts that are constantly moving and evolving. Parts that are connected to each other in ways that we are yet to understand.

It is only natural then that we don't have solutions to all the problems when some parts in this machinery don't function appropriately. While new research in modern medicine continues to fascinate us, there is another body of work that is equally mesmerising and can be used as a handy tool to find relief from at least some of our health issues—physical and mental. Ancient Indian scriptures provide a key to these tools. One such tool is pranayama, what we can loosely translate to breathing techniques.

THREE

KNOWLEDGE FROM SCRIPTURES

The earliest reference to pranayama is found in Vedic literature, dating back to before 1500 BC. At that time, pranayama was practised mainly as a part of religious ceremonies when the breath was held while reciting mantras in the mind. This was done to control the wavering mind, which made the mantra recitation more fruitful.

The most important milestone in the evolution of pranayama came when Rishi Patanjali (300 BC), through his *Yoga Sutras* described pranayama as a psycho-physiological practice, and a technique that led to mastery over the mind, *manojaya*. He acknowledged that the manipulation of the breath had a great physiological and psychological effect that could be utilised to improve the health of the mind-body complex.

Pranayama techniques were later harnessed and classified in the Hatha Yogic tradition (1000–1700 AD). The deliberate stopping of breath, *kumbhaka*, became the most important component of pranayama, so much so that the word *kumbhaka* was used as a synonym for pranayama.

In this tradition, methods of regulating the breath evolved using

- *bandhas*, internal body locks;
- *kriyas* like *kapalabhati* and *bhastrika*; and
- *mudras*, hand and finger positions for directing *prana*.

Details about the phases of breathing, their speed and ratios, and types and techniques of retention of breath, were added at this time.

Ancient Indian scripture understood anatomy and physiology a little differently from modern medicine. Again, while the knowledge is vast and deep, we offer only a glimpse of the portions that pertain to understanding pranayama. Various yogis conceptualised and categorised aspects of the human body in different ways. A study of the scriptures reveals four main categorisation methodologies. However, each model is connected to the other in one way or the other, and none of them can be considered independently.

By their very nature—and especially because the content of these theories is not always discernible to the eye or even under a microscope—they might sound abstract to some. Fortunately, the benefits derived from the underlying concepts do not depend on how much or how little we understand them—just like pressing a switch turns the relevant bulb on, whether or not the person pressing the switch understands how electricity works.

I suggest that you read the brief description that follows to imagine a world within us that holds potential and possibilities beyond our understanding. The hope is that this quick summary will allow you to understand why yogis pursued this line of thought.

THE MAIN MODELS OF ANATOMY AS PER SCRIPTURES

There's a world beyond what meets the eye.

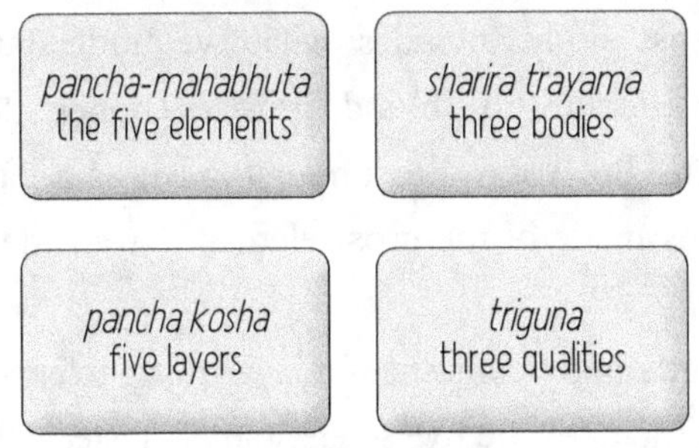

Our energy system: The main models of anatomy as per Indian scriptures

PANCHA-MAHABHUTA: THE FIVE ELEMENTS

The *pancha-mahabhuta* categorisation believes that everything about the body consists of one or more of the five elements—space, air, fire, water, and earth. The origin and culmination of everything in the world and thus, the human body is from and into these elements. Each element exists in varying degrees in all of nature's creation.

Also known as *pancha tatva*, this theory assigns each of these elements to various systems in the body. For instance, the five sensory organs and five main senses are related to the five different elements. Likewise, each element is associated with each of the five fingers in one hand.

SHARIRA TRAYAMA: THREE BODIES

In this model, the human body is conceptualised as having three parts, each of which is called a body itself—the gross body, the subtle body, and the causal body.

The gross body includes what we understand from modern medicine too—blood, muscles, bones, fluids, fat, marrow, etc. But yogis also understood it as a part of the body that is made of the gross elements from the *pancha-mahabhuta*.

The subtle body consists of a layer not perceivable to us directly. It includes the five senses (smell, taste, sight, touch and sound) to absorb input from the external world; the five action organs (hands, legs, speech, anus and genitals) to produce output into the outer world; the five *pranas* or energies that control the input and output within the body, and the four internal organs (mind, intellect, memory and ego) that form the mind space.

The causal body is even subtler than the subtle body. It is the seed that has the potential to shape the subtle and gross bodies. This body manifests itself from its seed form when it has a conducive environment. It also becomes the destination for the gross and subtle bodies when it is time for them to dissolve.

PANCHA KOSHA: FIVE LAYERS

The body is perceived as having five layers according to the *pancha kosha* understanding of the human body—the physical, vital energy, mental, wisdom and bliss layers. This correlates to the *sharira trayama* model in the sense that the physical layer can be thought of as the gross body. The other four layers are part of the subtle body. Within the fifth layer is the causal body. It would be a folly to think of these layers as separate entities. They intermingle and interconnect to make our body function as a holistic system.

In some sense, each cell can be thought of as having these five layers. After all, as the cells multiply, each cell has the intelligence to know what it is supposed to become, whether it is hand or hair, colon or heart, blood or marrow. Such intelligence needs input from all five layers to manifest in the appropriate physical form.

The vital energy layer, or the *pranamaya kosha*, is the most relevant to our discussion in this book. This connecting layer between the subtler layers of the body and the gross body has the potential to impact our being in both positive and negative ways. Pranayama is a set of techniques to control this energy and channel it in a positive direction. We will discuss the energy channels and hubs in a bit.

TRIGUNA: THREE QUALITIES

This understanding of anatomy believes that the human body has three categories of qualities—relatively negative ones such as laziness and materialism; high-energy ones such as anger and euphoria; and harmonious ones such as balance and joy. Each body is believed to have all three qualities in varying degrees.

With this basic understanding, let us take a look at the aspect that is most relevant to us—*prana*.

OUR ENERGY SYSTEM

The mystical *prana* and its ways can and must be understood.

One of the main underlying concepts in each of the models above is the concept of vital energy, the pathways it moves through and the hubs that it is concentrated at. These are *prana*, *nadi*s, and *chakra*s, respectively.

It is important to realise here that a lot of the ancient study had the spiritual aim of *moksha* or liberation—liberation from the pain and suffering that binds us to this earth; liberation from the cycle of birth, death, and rebirth; liberation so that we can know, truly know, that everything in the world has just one origin and culmination.

Like many yoga practitioners, I consider this spiritual goal a destination that is a little distant. The path is difficult and requires impenetrable focus, to put it mildly. Yet, as I know from my own journey, the application of this knowledge brings relief from physiological ailments such as psoriasis. And ironically enough, the side-effect is spiritual growth. How that came to be, requires us to delve a little deeper into how the energy system is said to work.

PRANA: OUR VITAL ENERGY

The *prana* in pranayama is often equated to breath. But, breath actually is only a medium to control *prana*, a subtler aspect of our existence. A closer translation of *prana* would be energy—the energy that we say is low when we are tired or sad, the energy that we are full of when we are pumped up or ecstatic, the energy that seems harmonious when we are content or joyous.

Another way to make the abstract facet of *prana* approachable is to consider the body at the time of death. The physical body does not disappear at death, but the energy that runs it leaves.

While the gross organs and limbs continue to exist, they stop functioning. The subtle layer of the body that makes the organs function has left the body. However, when these organs from the dead body are transplanted into the body of a person with the subtle body alive, the same organs begin to function. This aspect of the subtle body, this energy, this *prana* is essential for our existence. This is our vital energy.

The word *prana* from ancient Indian scriptures is considered the first energy–'*pra*' means first, and '*na* is the smallest unit of energy. All aspects and levels of creation manifest out of this first unit of energy. *Prana* is the primal or atomic beginning of the flow of energy from which emerge all other forms of energy.

All that vibrates in the universe is considered a form of *prana*—light, heat, sound, magnetism, gravity, electricity, power, vigour, and so on. Unfortunately, it has not yet been measured by existing scientific tools and methodologies. But, with our technological advances, the discovery doesn't seem out of reach. Even today, we can understand change in patterns by studying ECG[1], EEG[2] and EMG[3], even if the changes cannot be quantified.

Meanwhile, it is indeed this energy that is observed in the systolic and diastolic actions of the pumping heart, through the inhalations and exhalations of respiration, within the digestion and absorption of food, and in the excretion of urine and faeces.

Moreover, *prana* is not just our physical energy. It is also the subtler mental energy where the mind gathers information. It is the intellectual energy where information is examined and filtered.

Yogic philosophy believes that the stronger this life force is within us, the better we are and feel. A balance in the *prana* brings clarity of mind that makes decision-making easier and more efficient. Emotions, too, are steadier with a healthy flow of *prana* in the body.

FORMS OF *PRANA*

As per ancient Indian texts, *prana* is said to transform into various powers in the body for carrying out different

---

[1] ECG: Electrocardiogram measures electric activity of your heart.
[2] EEG: Electroencephalogram measures electric activity in your brain.
[3] EMG: Electromyograph measures electric activity in your muscles and nerves.

functions. It has five major functional aspects that feel more active in specific regions of the body. These functional aspects of *prana* have been given different names according to the bodily functions with which they correspond.

Udana prana is said to operate in the head and neck regions and is responsible for speech, expression, comprehension and communication.

Prana prana corresponds to the functions in the chest region—the heart and the lungs.

Samana prana is located in the central region of the body's trunk between the rib cage and the navel. It controls the digestive organs and their secretions and is responsible for the digestion and assimilation of nutrients.

Apana prana is found in the lower abdomen region and the pelvic region between the navel and the perineum. It controls the kidneys, the bowels, the bladder, the excretory and the reproductive organs. It is responsible for all expulsion in the body from gas, urine, faeces, and menstrual flow to the foetus at the time of birth.

Vyana prana exists throughout the body. It regulates all the muscular movements in the body through the nervous system.

Of course, all the forms of *prana* interact with each other and are co-dependent. The central idea is to maintain balance amongst them for a healthy body.

NADIS: THE ENERGY NETWORK

Prana is said to use specific channels to move through the body. These channels are known as *nadis*. The word *nadi* means 'river' or 'channel'. These *nadis* carry the flowing currents of energy to reach different areas in the body.

There is an intricate network of *nadis* all over the body, estimated at well over 72,000 by yogis. Counts in some texts add up to over 300,000. This network is similar to the network of nerves or blood vessels. Just like nerves carry impulses, and vessels ferry blood, *nadis* transmit *prana*. However, this is only a rough analogy.

Not all *nadis* are operational at all times. Some of them lie dormant until certain triggers awaken them. Also, more often than not, *nadis* are blocked for one reason or another. This hampers the free flow of *prana*, disrupting the normal functioning of body parts. If the obstruction lasts long, diseases can emerge.

THE THREE MAIN *NADIS*

Among the thousands of *nadis*, there are three very powerful channels which, when sufficiently unclogged, can promote growth on all three planes—physical, mental and spiritual, allowing us to reach higher levels of awareness. This leads to higher consciousness, which is a pre-requisite for attaining the true aim—liberation. These channels are *ida, pingala* and *sushumna.*

The configuration of these three *nadis* can be seen in ancient scriptures. Astonishing as it is, this is how they are also represented in the figure of Caduceus from ancient Greece. This figure is the universal symbol of medicine today. The central rod is symbolic of the spinal canal through which the central *nadi, sushumna,* runs. The *ida* and the *pingala nadis* are represented in the Caduceus by the two entwined snakes with their origins at the spinal base, moving up in a spiral formation, crossing at various points along the central rod.

The *ida* originates from the left side of the base of the spine and transverses spirally upwards to reach the roof of the left nostril. It is said to control all the activities that are anabolic or constructive in nature, activities that conserve energy and give a cooling effect to the body.

The *pingala* rises from the right side of the base of the spine and reaches the roof of the right nostril. It is said to control the activities of the body that consume energy and generate heat in the body.

Thus the *ida* and the *pingala* have opposite functions. What one can accelerate, the other can slow down. Ancient seers held that when *ida* and *pingala* are active together, the *sushumna* is triggered. This allows even and rhythmic mental and physical energy patterns leading to inner harmony.

CHAKRAS: THE ENERGY HUBS

Yogis' practical and systemic view of energy includes centres of *prana*, known as *chakra*s. The *prana* network is fuelled by these chakras that are high-powered vortices of energy. They receive *prana* from the outer world in the form of food, water, breath, and even good vibes and use it for the functioning of various organs and parts of the body.

While our body has many *chakra*s, seven of them are said to be of greater importance. Every individual is said to be most active at one chakra level or another, depending on their life situation and where they are in their spiritual journey.

Mooladhara chakra, the base or root chakra, is located in the region between the genitals and the anus. It relates to baser instincts such as security and survival. This chakra is the lowest of all chakras and is the seat of primal energy.

Swadhisthana chakra, or the sacral chakra, is found in the groin area and is associated with base emotions, sexuality and creativity. This chakra is the hub of sexual energy.

Manipura chakra, or the solar plexus chakra, is in the navel area and corresponds to the transition from the base to the higher emotions. It plays a role in assimilation and digestion.

These three levels of consciousness prevail throughout the animal kingdom. Much of society's ills can be considered a result of an imbalance in these chakras. The biggest step in human development is an ascent from this level of consciousness to a higher level through the other four chakras.

Anahata chakra, or the heart chakra is located in the chest area. It concerns itself with higher emotion, compassion, love, equilibrium, and well-being. It operates the immune system.

Vishuddhi chakra, or the throat chakra, is situated, as is obvious, in the throat area and relates to communication. It is said to be the location of intuitive skills.

Ajna chakra, or the third eye chakra, is located at the centre of the brain. *Ajna* is the chakra of awareness and enlightenment. It is the centre of wisdom that allows one to see beyond the polarities of right and wrong.

Sahasrara chakra, or the crown chakra, is located at the top-most part of the head. Some schools even believe it to be floating slightly above the head. This is the chakra of consciousness, the master chakra that controls all the others.

For holistic growth and harmony, all *chakras* are equally important. However, every individual might have some dominant *chakras* that establish their personality. As time goes by, this *chakra* may lose its dominance, and some others may gain importance, depending on the changes in one's life.

Again, each energy hub can go out of balance when the body doesn't receive *prana* in adequate quantity and quality. In turn, this creates a block and whatever *prana* exists is unable to circulate freely. This leads to distress, diseases and lack of mind-body integrity, which doesn't allow for

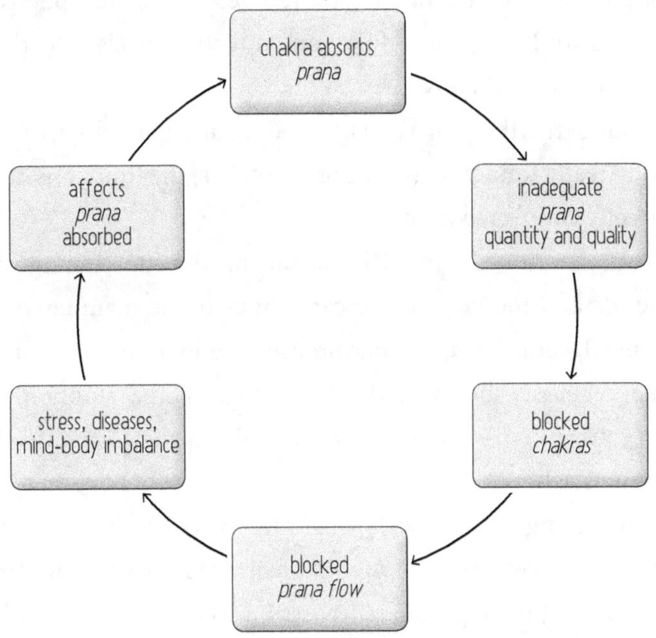

Chakras: The energy hubs

appropriate absorption of *prana*. And so continues the circle.

PHYSIOLOGY MEETS PHILOSOPHY: THE BODY-ENERGY CONNECT

It is all connected.

NADIS

The *ida nadi*, also known as the moon channel is associated with cooling the body down. This translates to lowering blood pressure and heart rate, recovery of dilated pupils, etc. As we know, these functions directly correlate to the functioning of the PNS.

Similarly, the *pingala nadi* or the sun channel gets the body ready for action—fight or flight. Yes, the functions are directly connected to the SNS.

As mentioned earlier, by balancing the functioning of the *ida* and the *pingala*, we can stimulate the main energy channel, *sushumna*, to harmonise bodily functions. Just like a balance between the two wings of the autonomic nervous system—the SNS and PNS—brings us to a state of homeostasis.

Breathing techniques, which we will discuss in later chapters, reveal that the *ida nadi* corresponds with airflow dominating through the left nostril, while the *pingala nadi* is associated with the airflow dominating the right nostril.

When airflow dominates through the right nostril, it is found to correlate with greater activity in the left hemisphere of the brain and vice versa.

It only seems natural that the correlation between *nadis* and the nervous system will lead us to a correlation between chakras and some parts of the physical body. Surely enough, it does.

CHAKRAS

More specifically, the *chakra* system manifests itself in the physical body through the neuro-endocrine system—the nervous system and the endocrine system.

You would recall, the nervous system, through the wide network of nerves and the endocrine system through chemical regulators called hormones, exert control over all our physical, mental, behavioural and emotional functions. If either of these two fail, the body gets jeopardised.

It is believed that *chakras* correspond to the autonomic nerve plexuses and endocrine glands. The SNS arises from that part of the spinal cord, which is in the chest and the lower back areas. The PNS from the brain and the tail bone region of the spinal cord. Together, they create a network of plexuses that link physiologically with the endocrine system. Lo and behold, the main *chakras* are located around these plexuses and glands.

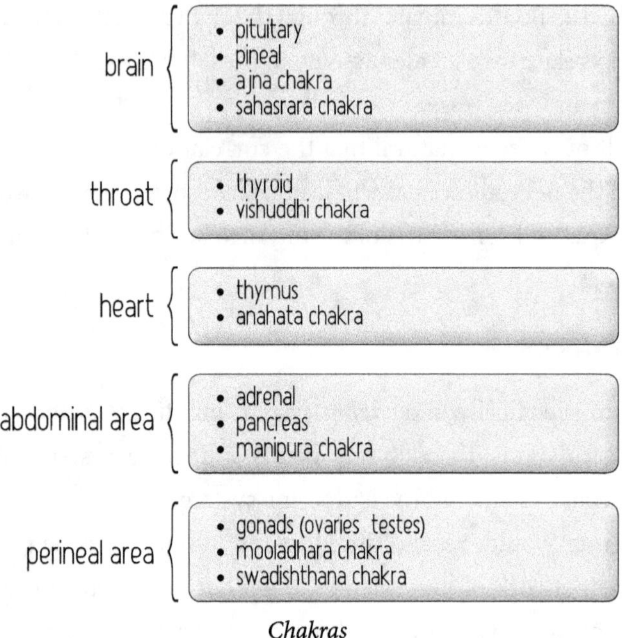

Chakras

Mooladhara chakra: Although no endocrine organ is present here, it is said to relate to the inner adrenal glands, the adrenal medulla, responsible for the fight-or-flight response when survival is under threat.

Swadhisthana chakra correlates to the sacral plexus, which is located at the base of the spine at the level of the tail bone and the pubis. The ovaries and testes are found in this area.

Manipura chakra is in line with the solar plexus, where the adrenal and pancreas glands lie.

Anahata chakra is around the cardiac plexus area, which is where the thymus gland is located.

Vishuddhi chakra is in the throat region, which is also where the laryngeal plexus is situated. The thyroid gland is also in this area.

Ajna chakra is located at the top of the spinal cord where the three major *nadis* meet, in the mid-brain area. This is where the all-important pineal gland is situated.

Sahasrara chakra is the centre and relates to the pineal gland and the cerebral cortex.

MODERN MEDICINE MEETS ANCIENT WISDOM

We are heading towards the intersection of technique and proof.

With this basic knowledge at our disposal, it is now becoming clearer that we have two extremely powerful tools at our disposal. Modern medicine deals with aspects of the disease that are caused by externalities. The methods used—from antibiotics to surgery—provide immediate relief.

This is where ancient yogic wisdom related to *prana* can come into play and work on internal imbalances that could be the root cause of said disease. Of course, this can be used as a preventive tool to begin with, and also help mitigate or reduce chances of a relapse or recurrence of the disease. When it cannot do any of that, it can muster the mental strength required to deal with the situation. Who can deny that physical ailments take a toll on mental health?

It is important to note that a major portion of *prana* is used up by the body for its routine processes such as digestion, elimination, sexual activity, and repair and maintenance. The energy left after these activities is used by the mind to feel, comprehend, analyse, learn, experience and reflect.

If the energy is in short supply, the mind suffers because routine processes are prioritised. This, however, leads to lethargy, lack of alertness, etc.

Disease occurs when the energy is in constant short supply. Which part of the body suffers depends on individual tendencies. If this involves a small area, it gives rise to pain. If it extends over a larger area or for a longer duration, it then manifests as a disease. Total exhaustion of this energy is death.

PRANA MEETS BREATH

Why are we low in energy or *prana*? It is mainly due to faulty and ineffective breathing habits, chronic stress and its effect on our minds.

Prana flow is regulated at and by energy hubs that are located near plexuses of the nervous system and important endocrine glands. Breath is a bodily function that is involuntary and can be controlled voluntarily—two aspects of the nervous system. The nervous system meets at the hypothalamus, which connects to the pineal gland of the endocrine system.

We, therefore, can use our breaths to influence the nervous and endocrine systems. By virtue of their location, they interact with the *prana* system. *Prana* can influence the nervous and endocrine systems. Miraculously enough, we can participate in our health.

MIND AND BREATH

Our mental state affects our breath. When we are excited, the breath becomes quicker, and when we are calm and relaxed, it is quieter. Any activity that requires total concentration will also control our breath. For example, while threading a needle, our breath stops for a moment; the thought process also stops for a few seconds as the mind is completely focused and engaged.

Fortunately, the reverse is true too. We can change our breath to influence the mind. We can voluntarily tackle our mind and our emotions through the breath, which works with *prana*. Of course, not all problems can be solved completely. But, we can certainly work on the quantity and quality of our responses to the problems.

Participating in our health is miraculously possible.

Through pranayama—the science of the control of *prana* or the life force—one uses the breath to manage the amount, flow and distribution of energy to both the body and the mind. This is the aim of this book—breath-management for both body-management and mind-management.

HOW DO
WE GET
THERE

FOUR

TAKING CONTROL OF OUR HEALTH

Modern medicine has made our lives longer and better to a great extent. Breathing practices can make the quality of our lives even better. Also, these techniques allow us to better manage the suffering we live with because of our ailment. Further, consistent practice can take our state of mind, irrespective of the state of the body, beyond what we could have imagined—to a place of acceptance and peace.

At a gross level, we have understood that our breaths are the connectors between our physical body and the inner world within. Working on the physical aspects of breathing corrects the imbalances in the working of the bodily organs and alters the internal state of affairs.

And we have ample to work with. Life begins with a breath, usually accompanied by a sound, as we emerge as babies from the womb. We don't need anyone to teach us how to breathe, and we continue to do it all our lives. Approximately, we inhale and exhale sixteen times a minute, that is 21,600 times in a day.

Each of the seventy-five trillion cells in our body absorb the oxygen we breathe in, and by the process of metabolism, produce the carbon dioxide that we breathe out. Unsurprisingly then, it affects our sleep, memory, concentration and our energy levels. Indeed, every aspect of our personality depends on our breath.

And yet, most of us take our breath for granted; we breathe merely to survive. This is as much a product of our chronically stressful lifestyle as it is of us being ignorant of the importance of our breaths. We are not really aware of our breathing, let alone checking if we are breathing correctly.

As a result, we neither take in sufficient oxygen nor do we eliminate enough carbon dioxide. This build-up leads to generalised physical tension, reduced vitality, emotional instability, confused thought processes, depleted energy, premature ageing, poorly functioning immune system, sleep disorders, stomach upsets, muscle cramps, anxiety, dizziness, chest pains, and palpitations—to name a few.

Fortunately, just like correcting your diet can affect required changes for a healthy body, correct breathing too can do the same. Using our conscious will, we can alter our breathing to deepen it, slow it down, make it rhythmic and allow it to flow freely. This is called 'conscious breathing'.

To reiterate a point made in an earlier chapter, consider this. Can we use our free will to command our digestive system to digest food faster? Can we request the kidneys to filter out the urine slower so that we can enjoy undisturbed sleep? No. Breathing, on the other hand, can be instantaneously controlled or manipulated using our conscious will. And this control over our breath can be used as a tool to regulate all other vital functions like digestion and metabolism, as well as control the mind.

"HOW" IS MORE IMPORTANT THAN "WHAT"

**Our breath's quality guides our life's quality.
No exaggeration.**

Becoming aware of our breath is half the job done. Of course, awareness is not easy to come by and requires practice and patience. However, it is not out of reach, especially when you know what you are doing. Once you know how to and practise consistently, you are likely to fall into the correct pattern.

Merely watching and focusing on our respiration and following its natural rhythm deepens our breath automatically. When we begin, though, we will realise that our automatic breathing is not the most efficient. There are a few aspects that need slight modification or correction. We will take these up in turn.

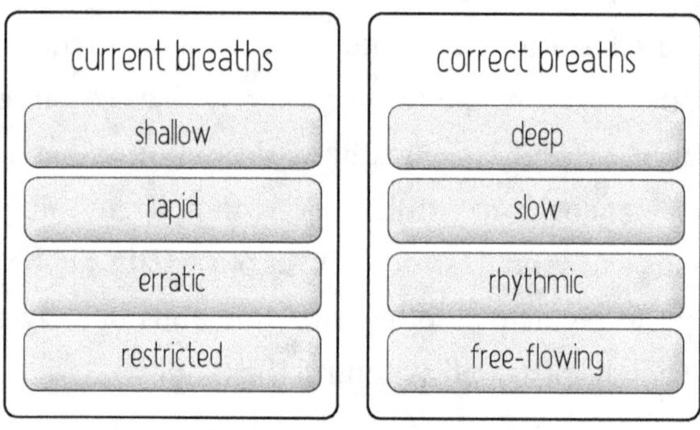

How we breathe is important

SHALLOW BREATHING

As new-born babies, we breathe with our abdomen. Our lower belly rises and falls with each breath. As we grow older, we, for one reason or another, 'hold ourselves in'. This could be our mechanism to protect ourselves from hurtful comments, emotional knocks, and confusing messages. This 'holding' starts taking the form of held breaths. With advancing age, chronic stress pushes our muscles into a state of constant tension, preventing the respiratory muscles from functioning fully. Sustained pressure in the back muscles and the shoulders due to wrong posture and stress compromise our breathing.

Consequently, our breathing becomes shallower, proceeding from what is called 'abdominal breathing' to 'chest breathing' and then to 'shoulder breathing'. The last is the most common kind of breathing. It is restricted to the collarbone and the shoulders and reaches at most to mid-chest level. In this type of breathing, the lower parts of the lungs are practically unventilated. There is no exchange of air in the area, and the stale air accumulates in the lungs. This is the least desirable form of breathing as it prevents us from taking in sufficient oxygen and eliminating enough carbon dioxide.

As a result, a toxic build-up occurs in the body, leading to reduced vitality, premature ageing, and a poor immune system. Shoulder breathing is so common that it is accepted as the norm. However, it often leads to physical tension, digestive disorders, lethargy, emotional instability, a confused thought process, and concomitant stress. Lack of sufficient oxygen is also a major contributing factor in heart disease, cancer and paralytic stroke.

Older people or those who are seriously ill have very shallow and quick breaths with shoulders rising and falling at every breath. The shallowest breathing is 'throat breathing'. When breathing becomes shallower than this, a person dies.

REVERSE BREATHING

The habit formed out of being constantly anxious and fearful continues. As we experience fear, our automatic response is to inhale and hold our breath. The belly gets sucked in at the same time. This is the exact opposite of what we would do if we were breathing normally. We then hold our breath until the danger passes. After that, quickly and with an outward sigh, we release both the breath and the belly outwards.

Therefore, our automatic response of taking a breath in and pulling our belly in when under stress is contrary to our body's natural flow. Exhalations, too, are incomplete because we let out a sigh when the pressure passes and let our belly bulge out too. The outward movement of the abdomen prevents proper emptying of the lungs.

CURTAILED EXHALATIONS

Exhalation is a crucial part of the breathing process. Not only do the lungs expel carbon dioxide when we exhale, but our nervous system also gets a chance to let the parasympathetic part of it function. In everyday life, of course, our exhalations are short.

Interestingly, this might continue when we breathe consciously, too, especially in the beginning. In our attempt to breathe in deeply, we breathe out quickly, cutting our exhalations short. Taking in a few deep breaths with sharp exhalations is not a quick fix.

SLIMMER'S BREATH

Some people habitually hold in their abdominal muscles to appear slimmer. This tension obstructs the breathing process, making it shallow and restricted. Not only do the cells get deprived of oxygen, but the abdominal organs too do not get a chance to freely move back into place on exhalation.

SINGLE NOSTRIL DOMINATION

Try this simple experiment. Breathe through one nostril at a time instead of both as one unit. Do this by blocking one nostril with your finger and observe the flow in the other for a few breaths. Repeat with the other nostril. You will notice that one nostril is generally more open than the other. If you repeat this experiment at different times of the day, you will see that sometimes one side is clear and at other times, for no apparent reason, it seems blocked. You will observe that this is so even when you may not be suffering from any allergy or cold.

This is actually a regular cyclical phenomenon occurring throughout the day. Congestion of the nostril lining changes from one nostril to the other every 1.5-2 hours. This rhythm which most of us are unaware of, is called the nasal cycle.

The nostrils are richly endowed with twenty times

more autonomic nerve fibres, which connect them to the hypothalamus in the brain. As you would recall, the hypothalamus, along with the ANS, controls innumerable physiological functions and emotional states.

The dominance of sympathetic activity on one side narrows the blood vessels, allowing greater airflow through the nostrils. At this time, the other nostril exhibits a simultaneous dominance of the parasympathetic activity, causing local swelling and thus a restricted airflow.

While these are natural patterns, our lifestyle and activities disturb the pattern, and one nostril or one side of respiration ends up being used more than the other. This could be because of the changing temperature in the environment, our posture and physical state, or our mental state.

Ancient yoga gurus observed that this asymmetric breathing also governs many activities of the body, such as the functioning of the internal organs, the onset of disease, and the equanimity or instability of the mind. Scriptures on Swara Yoga like the *Shiva Swarodaya* claim that the modes of mental activity too, depend on which nostril is dominant or most open to airflow.

The texts also propound that an abnormally long dominance of one nostril is an indication of physical or mental ill health.

- If the right nostril is overly dominant, the result is mental and nervous disturbances.
- If the left nostril is overly dominant, the result is fatigue and reduced energy levels.

This correlates well with our physiological understanding of the body. Continuous dominance by a particular nostril signifies an imbalance between the active SNS (*pingala nadi*) and the healing PNS (*ida nadi*). When the ability of the body to balance gets deranged, it results in ill health and disease.

BODY, MIND AND BREATH

Every breath we take, indeed, affects every move we make.

STRESS, FATIGUE AND OUR BREATHS

Are you constantly tired? Do you feel drained out by midday? Do you take vitamin supplements? Subject yourself to a battery of tests, only to get normal results that do not explain the fatigue? Is it all just in your mind? The answer is simple, if not obvious. Poor quality of breathing is the underlying cause of many of your symptoms. This includes muscle cramps, chest pains, premenstrual tensions and headaches.

It is the same principle that we began with. When we are chronically in a state of stress, we tax our SNS. This leads to 'more-than-what-it-should-be' levels of heart rate, blood pressure, muscular tension, blood sugar level, etc.—constantly. This affects us on a deeper physical and emotional level. When we cannot cope further, the body breaks down, and we are struck down with all kinds of illnesses.

Stress not only alters our emotional and mental states but also our breathing. When we are agitated, our breathing pattern becomes erratic: we take in a breath, hold it and then let go quickly. The same is the case when we are full of tension. Our breathing becomes irregular and shallow.

Thoughts produce stress, too. Thoughts need energy to come and go. At times the mind is 'racing' while at other times we are 'too tired to think'. As adults, we have learnt to control our speech and breathing. We handle our daily tensions by somehow holding our breath and controlling our thoughts. But thoughts rarely stay under control, and they can be chaotic. They cause stress in our breathing and spill out in the form of physical illness.

This arrhythmic, rapid, chest-level, sharp breathing, in turn, keeps the body and mind agitated, leading to a circle of stress and non-effective breathing. And yet, this cycle itself can help us fix what is broken and improve what is not broken.

WELL-BEING AND OUR BREATHS

Nature has provided a potent tool to combat the harmful effects of stress—our PNS. If we understand and implement techniques to make it function as necessary, we can use this gift of nature. Some methods include good quality and quantity of sleep, relaxation, pranayama, meditation, music, soft emotions, love, compassion, forgiveness and acceptance.

Conscious breathing holds an exceptional place here. Our breath is the first to get affected by stress. But, with our breathing, we can influence our nervous system, transform our mental, emotional and even physical health, and maintain well-being. How we breathe and how much we give ourselves a chance to breathe consciously every day can strongly influence our health. Thus, we can improve our stress responses by honing our skills to regulate our breath.

Taking a breath with awareness is like combing the energy in and around us. It is like getting up in the morning with dishevelled hair. And as we brush and smooth the hair down, we untangle the knots. Breathing does more or less the same thing to our state of mind. With deep inhalations and exhalations, we align or 'comb' the energy around us.

Pranayama, the yogic breathing practices, involve slow diaphragmatic breathing. They are known to have shifted the basal autonomic balance to the parasympathetic direction. This reduces the adverse psycho-physiological and psychological effects of chronic stress and reactivity in stressful situations. The stress-reducing benefits of slow, deep, diaphragmatic breathing in patients with heart disease, hypertension and asthma, have made these breathing practices a valuable component of many integrated treatment programmes.

REVERSING INEFFECTIVE HABITS

To err is human. To self-correct is divine.

The first step, then, is to correct our breathing patterns. The step even before that is to know our current breathing pattern. So, before we learn any special breathing exercises, we should know if we are breathing correctly. And, if we are not, we should know how to correct it.

SIT RIGHT OR LIE DOWN

To start off on this journey, we have to know how to sit correctly. While practising any breathing exercise, the spine must be kept straight. This allows for the free flow of air. A hunched or collapsed spine impedes this flow. At the same time, in our enthusiasm to lengthen the spine at the chest area, we do not want to over-arch our lower back either.

While posture itself is a nuanced topic, to keep ourselves on the topic, we will refrain from going into those details.

Sitting straight means aligning and balancing the spine along a vertical axis ascending from the base to the skull. However, many of us may also find it difficult to sit in a meditative pose for a long period because we are not habituated to sitting in the recommended cross-legged postures. If bodily discomfort becomes a reason for distraction, we do not get any benefit out of the practice of pranayama. The mind gets diverted towards the discomfort instead of enjoying the subtle effects of pranayama.

The aim is not to sit in a complicated posture, but to sit so comfortably that one forgets the body and can delve deep into the subtler aspects. Posture and sitting problems should not be a reason for avoiding the practice of pranayama. Distortions of the spine are not only uncomfortable, but on a very subtle level, block the flow of energy. You can identify one of the ways in which your sitting posture begins to get distorted:

Rounded and hunched-up shoulders: It is difficult to straighten the upper back and expand the chest when the balls of the shoulders inadvertently curl forward.

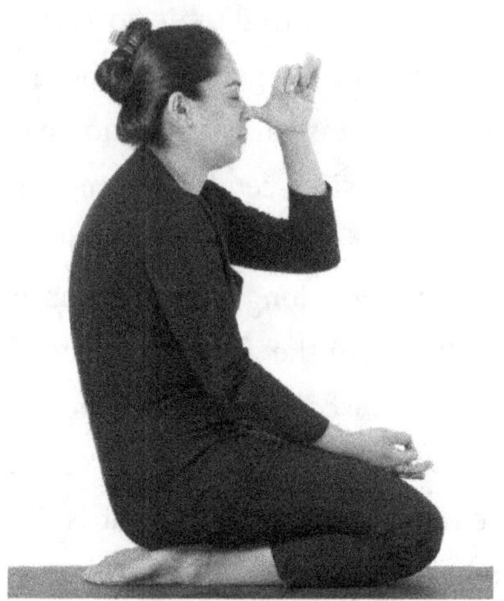

Vajrasana wrong with rounded back

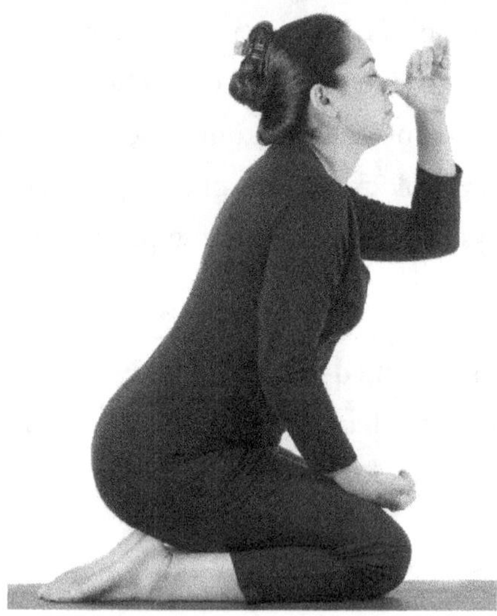

Vajrasana wrong with arched back

Stiff lower back or tight leg muscles: The natural curvature of the lower back gets distorted, collapsing the spine at the lower back. To counterbalance the feeling of falling backward because of this collapse, the upper back rounds and pushes forward. This leads to a stiff lower back and tight leg muscles.

Over-arched lower back: Some of us tend to push the pelvis forward, creating tension in the lower spine, the hips and even the neck. It can cause pain below the shoulder blades too.

Forward or backward lean: The head or even the entire body leans forward or backward because the muscles aren't trained to keep the shoulders, neck and head on top of the hips.

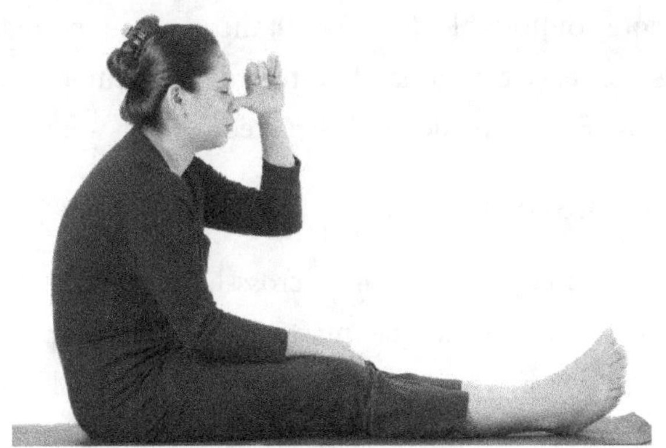

Wrong sitting on floor

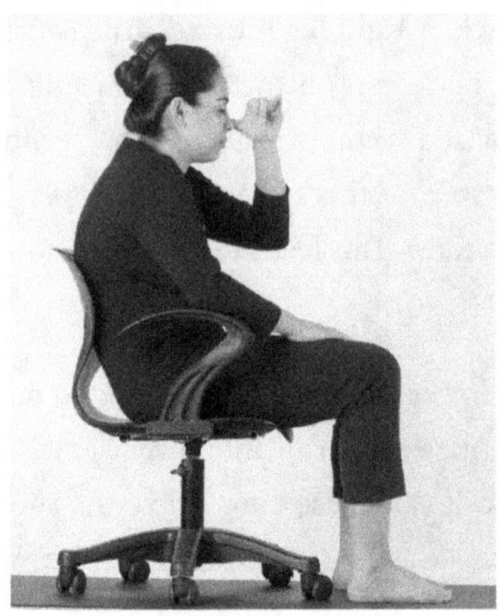

Wrong sitting on chair

The general principle is that the spine should be comfortably alert yet maintain its natural curves. We describe a few seated positions below and adjustments you could make to feel more comfortable. In all cases, the jaws are relaxed, the hands are relaxed in a hand gesture of your choice, unless otherwise recommended or instructed.

CROSS-LEGGED POSES

The scriptures describe 4-5 cross-legged postures for meditation. These can be mastered under the practical guidance of a yoga teacher: *padmasana* (full lotus), *ardhapadmasana* (half lotus), *siddhasana*, *swastikasana*, and *sukhasana* (simple cross-legged sitting). If you are a regular practitioner, you can pick the posture that you are most comfortable with and hold it without moving a lot. If you are not familiar with the postures, sit in a simple cross-legged posture. The aim is to sit with ease and without any distractions.

Yogic belief proposes that the erect spine position offers the least resistance to pranic energy, which is awakened through meditation and travels up to the brain.

PHYSIOLOGICAL ADVANTAGES OF CROSS-LEGGED POSTURES

Cross-legged postures offer a broad, firm, triangular foundation to the spine, where the spine is erect and all the body parts are relaxed. These poses prevent the body from collapsing forward, stooping, or tilting to either side. The natural curves of the spine are maintained without distortion. The head, neck, chest and abdomen are in perfect alignment so that the muscles for respiration can move freely. Also, minimum energy is required to maintain the posture.

The brain doesn't have to work too hard to maintain balance. Gravity and anti-gravity muscles need not work hard to maintain the pose since the firm triangular base provided by the crossed legs is enough. Closing the eyes is also possible without losing balance.

Moreover, the nervous system too is under minimal stress, and the mind can be peaceful and relaxed, yet alert.

The pelvic region (the lower trunk) gets a rich supply of blood, resulting in the toning of the nerves coming from the sacral (the lower part of the spinal cord) region. This increases the balance towards the parasympathetic nervous system, thereby easing and releasing stress.

An erect spine allows all the physiological activities to continue smoothly. Physiology says that erect postures create a proper balance for the digestive organs, the heart and the lungs, which can then function at an optimum level.

The abdominal muscles, the diaphragm and the muscles in the chest are stressed minimally. Production of carbon dioxide is minimised, hence, the process of breathing is more efficient. The continuous movement of the diaphragm and the ribs does not disturb the meditative state as you progress in your practice.

Only the supine position, that is, the lying-down position, is more relaxed than the meditative position, but there is always a possibility of falling asleep in a horizontal position.

Put together, all of the above allow you to sit comfortably for a long time.

USE OF PROPS

Understandably, most of the cross-legged poses are difficult for beginners to maintain. As someone just starting off, you can sit in any comfortable sitting position of your choice. If your back tends to lean forward or backward, or you are slouching either in your upper back or lower back, place your hips halfway on a cushion. While the hips are on the cushion, only the top part of your thighs should be on the cushion. This elevation of your tailbone gives your lower spine space to become straighter.

If this elevation is not enough, you can use two cushions, a bolster, or even a small stool. In this case, if your knees tend to dangle, support them with other cushions. Yes, that is a lot of cushions, but remember, the idea is that you should be able to focus on your breath without distractions.

If you are fidgety or uncomfortable with props too, you can try some other sitting postures.

THUNDERBOLT POSE

Vajrasana or thunderbolt pose straightens your spine without letting your lower back over-arch. To get into the pose, you stand on your knees and then lower your hips on your heels. The feet make a V-shape with heels apart and the big toes touching each other.

If in a bit your knees start sensing discomfort, you can place a cushion above your calves and rest your thighs on the cushion. This makes the angle at the knees less acute, avoiding the uncomfortable torque. However, if you experience or are prone to acute/chronic knee pain, do not sit in this pose.

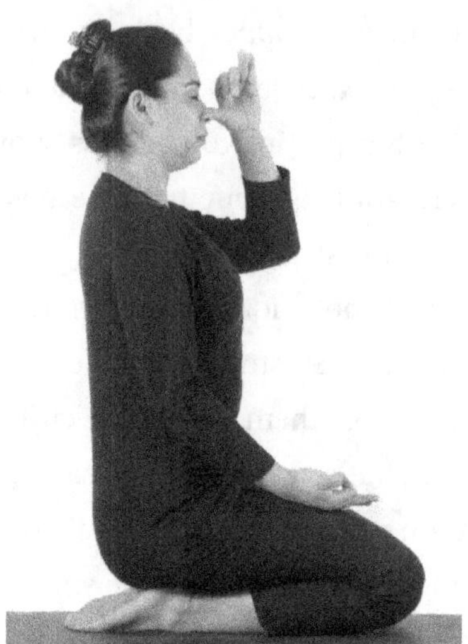

Vajrasana-correct posture

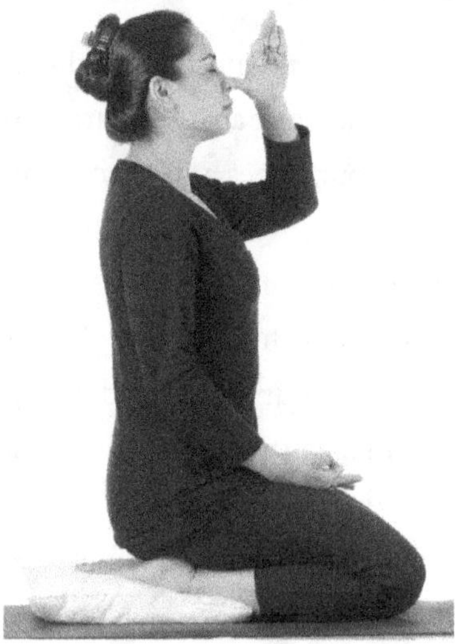

Vajrasana with one cushion

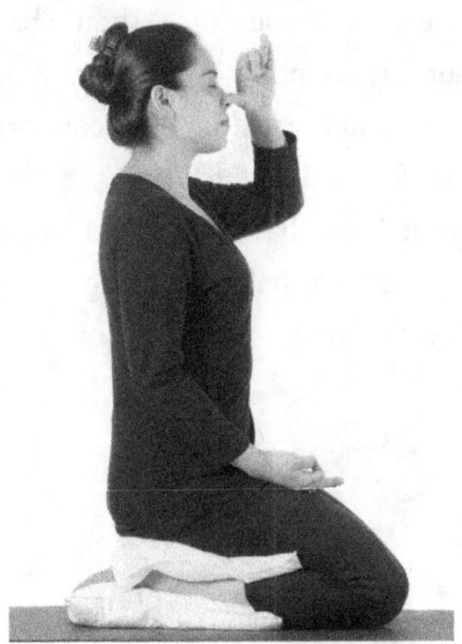

Vajrasana with two cushions

ON A CHAIR

If you cannot sit cross-legged for too long, it is okay to sit on a chair. This might be true if you have old injuries, or extreme stiffness of the knees, the hips or the back. This alternative will allow you to maintain a steady and comfortable posture with a straight spine.

Make sure the chair is firm. Keep a 90° or greater angle at your hip, between the thighs and the back. The height of the chair should be such that the hips are at a slightly higher level than the knees. As the thighs gently slope forward, the strain in the legs gets minimised.

Similarly, the angle at your knees should be 90° or more. Make sure your feet are not crossed. They shouldn't dangle either. Your feet should reach the floor comfortably. It is ok if you sit slightly forward on the chair.

Again, if your lower back still tends to collapse, place your hips on a cushion, half-way along its length to give your thighs a gentle slope.

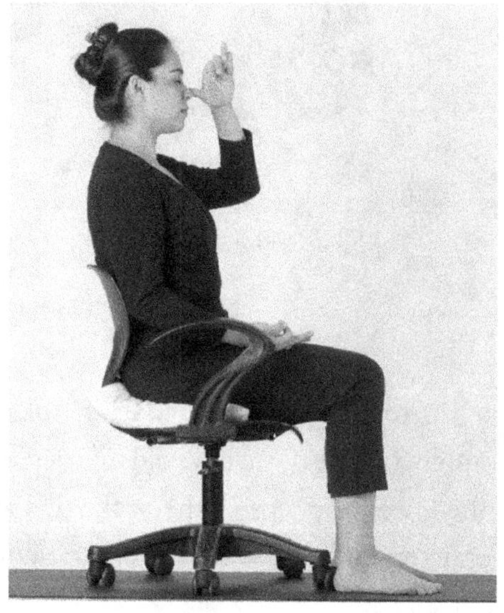

Correct sitting on chair with cushion

LIE ON BACK

If you cannot hold any sitting position comfortably, it is okay to lie down on the back with legs folded or straight, whichever is comfortable. Place a thin pillow below your head, such that your neck is in line with the spine.

If your lower back is over-arched when you straighten your legs, you can place a pillow or a bolster under your knees to flatten your lower back. While it is recommended that breathing practices be done while sitting down, almost all of them can be done lying down.

These postural guidelines should be followed for every pranayama/conscious breathing session, irrespective of how advanced your practice is.

CHECKING CURRENT BREATHING PATTERN

Identifying the current breathing pattern itself requires a certain quietude and awareness. It is okay if you are not able to recognise your pattern in one go. Give yourself time. Here are the things you should be careful about. They are in line with the common breathing patterns we discussed earlier.

Sit in a position of your choice and gently close your eyes. After a few breaths, start observing the movement of your breath. You are looking for the following patterns.

Shallow breathing: If your belly is not moving at all when you breathe, you are most likely a shallow breather. In all likelihood, only people who breathe with awareness all the time are deep breathers.

Reverse breathing: If your belly is moving, but you tend to

- suck or pull it in when asked to inhale or
- bloat it out when asked to exhale

you are a reverse breather.

On an average, 9 out of 10 people I have taught are reverse breathers. So, do not worry, you are not alone.

If you cannot make out the movement of your belly in coordination with your inhalation and exhalation, place your palm on your belly. If your palm moves out when you exhale and moves in when you inhale, you have identified your reverse breathing.

Curtailed exhalations: If you let out the air in a burst, your exhalations are shortened.

Slimmer's breath: If you tend to hold your belly in whether you are breathing in or out, you are a victim of slimmer's breath.

Single nostril domination: You can check for this after a few sessions. Once you have corrected your breaths for one or more of the above errors, you will be sufficiently aware to check for single nostril domination.

Follow this process every couple of hours for one or two days:

- Hold a mirror in front of your nostrils.

- Breathe out gently, without any manipulation, a few times.
- Observe the condensation of your breath on the mirror.
- It will be different on the left and right sides.
- The side that shows more condensation is the more active one.
- If you notice that one side is active a greater number of times over one or two days, you are breathing dominantly from that side.

CORRECTING ERRONEOUS BREATHING PATTERNS

If you have not identified any of the above errors, you are well on your path to conscious breathing. However, if you observe any of the above discrepancies, here are the guidelines for correcting them.

Do note that in any of the below corrections, even as you allow your belly to go out when you breathe in, do not allow it to bloat out completely. Such bloating will tend to pull your lower back forward, causing an unhealthy extra arch. So, when you let your belly inflate on an inhalation, allow it to stay half an inch inside its maximum bloating capacity.

SHALLOW AND REVERSE BREATHING

While just the act of observing often leads to the deepening of breaths to belly level, it might not always work. If this occurs, you can try one or more of these tips to deepen your breath. One tip might work better for you than others.

PALM ON BELLY

Place any one of your palms on your belly. Start with an exhalation. As you exhale, intentionally allow your palm to push your belly in. As you inhale, intentionally allow your palm to rise up with your belly.

VISUALISATION

Imagine that your lungs are balloons that you are filling up with air through your nostrils. As you breathe in, the lower parts of the balloon fill up, pushing the diaphragm down. This reduces the space available for your abdominal organs. So, make space for them by inflating the belly outward. As you breathe out, the air is let out of the balloons. The diaphragm moves back to its original position, making room for the abdominal organs to recede as well.

Take about 8-10 breaths till this becomes a natural pattern. Come back to it a couple of hours later. As is typical, you might observe that you have fallen back into your old habit. Take another 8-10 corrective breaths. Repeat this every couple of hours. Initially, you may have to concentrate hard. After a few attempts, you will feel the difference, and the body will begin to cooperate. In a few days, you will observe that your breathing pattern is more often correct than not.

AUTOMATIC CORRECTION IN LYING-DOWN POSITION

We breathe naturally and deeply while lying down or sleeping. Merely by lying down, our breaths correct themselves. So lie down, close your eyes, relax your body and observe your breaths. If you cannot observe directly, initially, you can place a book or your palm on the belly and follow it, moving up with an inhalation and down with an exhalation.

Focusing on the correct belly movement, gently turn to one side. Make sure you are still breathing comfortably and correctly. Gently sit up maintaining the breathing pattern.

CURTAILED EXHALATIONS

As you practise the above exercise, the exhalations automatically tend to become longer. It is possible that you are breathing correctly and deeply, and yet your exhalations are short. In such a case, focus on the first few seconds of your exhalation. We tend to sharply or quickly exhale in these first couple of seconds. Try to slow down the breath and allow as little air as possible to pass in these first two seconds. Once the first few seconds of exhalation are slower, the rest of the exhalation automatically slows down.

Be careful, though, not to exert yourself as you slow your exhalation down. It is something that comes with practice. And the practice should be guided by the comfort and effortlessness you feel while you are doing it.

SLIMMER'S BREATH

If you notice that you are holding your abdominal muscles tight even when you inhale, you keep yourself from taking a complete breath. The only way to correct this is to consciously let go of the over-tightness of the belly area during inhalations. Yes, like we mentioned earlier, you should not be expanding your belly out completely. At the same time, you should not be over-tightening your belly either. Balance is key, which comes with a gentle tone in the abdominal area.

SINGLE NOSTRIL DOMINATION

Do note that at any given time, breaths are known to be dominant in one nostril over the other. It is meant to change every 1.5-2 hours. Only and only if the same nostril dominates your breaths almost every time you check, would you correct the pattern.

Once you have identified the more dominant nostril, take deep and mindful breaths from the other side. So, inhale and exhale gently from the less dominant side to correct single nostril domination.

CONSCIOUS BREATHING

Our breath is our guide, our companion.

Once we have corrected the above patterns, we are ready to step into the deep and vast ocean of pranayama. A point well worth repeating is that your breath should be slow, deep, rhythmic and smooth-flowing. If we were to assign numbers, it would mean:

Slow: Each inhalation should take a minimum of four seconds. Each exhalation should take anywhere between four to eight seconds. The longer, the better. The ratio of inhalation to exhalation should be 1:2. So, irrespective of how many seconds you take to inhale, your exhalation should be at least as long and take double the length if possible. We will talk about this at great length in a bit.

Deep: Every exhalation should deflate the belly, pulling the navel in comfortably. Then the chest collapses, and shoulders relax. Every inhalation will fill up your belly owing to the descending diaphragm, pushing the navel out. It would then expand the chest laterally and fill the shoulders in a relaxed manner.

Rhythmic: Your inhalation to exhalation ratio would continue to be the same or improve, breath after breath. If a breath is shorter or shallower than the previous one, it could mean that you are exerting yourself beyond your capacity to extend the breath for longer. This is counter-productive. Strained breaths do no good. The remedy would be to reduce the length of your breath and try again.

Smooth-flowing: The breath should be subtle. No one sitting around you should notice that you are breathing any different. A sign that you are breathing smoothly is when you sense minimal-to-no movement of air around the tips of your nostrils. It is as if you want to cause as little disturbance to the environment around you. This becomes especially tricky when you are learning to count the number of seconds it takes you to breathe in and out. Often, the breath causes a jerk at every count. Once you become aware of it, it becomes easier to avoid the jerk. It is only a matter of practice.

Conscious breathing is closely related to the movement of the diaphragm, the dome-shaped muscular structure that separates the chest from the abdomen. When we breathe deeply, our diaphragm moves downward as we inhale and upward as we exhale. The more the diaphragm moves, the more our lungs can expand, which means that much more oxygen can be taken in, and more carbon dioxide is released with each breath.

Deep, conscious breathing can also be thought of as three-part breathing or sectional breathing. You fill and empty out the entire lung capacity. Begin with an exhalation.

For a slow, maximum exhalation, you would:

Step 1: Empty the upper chest to relax the shoulders.

Step 2: Once the middle and lower ribcages are drawn in, relax the chest area.

Step 3: When the abdomen is emptied, it gets pulled in.

Maximum inhalation would involve the breath being taken to:

Step 1: Expand the abdomen such that it is pushed out gently.

Step 2: The lower and middle ribcage can be observed in an expanding chest area.

Step 3: Finally, the upper ribcage expands and can be felt in the filling up of the shoulders. Be careful not to lift the top of the shoulders towards the ear, though.

We can go back to our balloon analogy. A balloon gets filled from the bottom up. When you release the air, it empties from the top first. Similarly, our lungs start filling from the lower part, the air proceeding upwards as we inhale. The emptying of the lungs begins from the upper part of the chest towards the lower parts.

To understand this coordination, place the right hand on the stomach and the left hand on the chest. You can practise this sitting, standing or lying down. Ensure that your breaths are slow, continuous, smooth and flowing, without any interruption. There should be no effort or strain.

Begin by exhaling completely through the nose. When the exhalation is complete, the stomach and the right hand placed on it, will move in towards the spine. The left hand would be drawn towards the middle of the chest, laterally.

Begin the inhalation by expanding the stomach area with the right hand still on it being pushed out. Allow the lower lungs to fill. Continue to inhale, allowing the lower ribcage to expand, moving the left palm slightly to the left. The upper chest will also fill up slowly.

Again, while exhaling, release the air from the upper chest to draw the hand back in place. Then the lower chest empties, and finally, the abdominal section comes in toward the spine.

Continue the slow and deep breaths for a few minutes, ending with an exhalation. If you feel tired, short of breath, or dizzy, go back to normal breathing for a while. You can try sectional breathing after a few breaths.

IMPORTANCE OF EXHALATIONS

As adults, our hurry-and-worry type of living leads to shallow and rapid breathing and curtailed exhalations. We have not only forgotten how to breathe correctly, but the ratio between our inhalations and exhalations, too, is quite erratic. As mentioned earlier, when we breathe optimally and in a relaxed way, the natural ratio of inhalation to exhalation is 1:2. This means that the exhalation is twice as long as the inhalation. So, if we inhale for two seconds, the exhalation should generally last about four seconds, without any discomfort. As you would expect, this doesn't hold true for most of us who do not breathe with awareness.

A complete and unrestricted exhalation is more vital than only a deep inhalation. It is during this exhalation that the relaxation response gets triggered. With a long and slow exhalation, the PNS is triggering the relaxation response. The smooth, quiet, relaxed and free-flowing breath, a product of mindful breathing, works on all bodily functions that are required to come back to normal from their stressed-out positions. Breathing this new, deeper way allows the heart to rest as the heart rate slows down, giving the heart more time to relax. It also produces a sense of stability and a positive feeling of security.

A good exhalation results naturally in a subsequent fuller and unforced inhalation. With regular practice, the breath becomes freer, steadier and deeper, without any conscious effort on our part.

Of course, you need to practise frequently and make it a part of your regular routine over the long term. At the same time, you should also acknowledge that each session might bring a new experience. The aim is to be aware and accept it for what it is. Therefore, don't ever force yourself to achieve the mentioned 1:2 ratio to progress more rapidly. Sooner or later, the body will react negatively to this forced way of breathing. Build your ratios up gradually because only then will the body adapt naturally, avoiding problems later.

BUILDING THE 1:2 RATIO

At first, only observe. Count the number of seconds taken to inhale and the number of seconds taken to exhale. Don't interfere or try to manipulate, just observe. In fact, begin each session with such non-judgemental observation. Then whatever the length of your inhalation, try to extend the exhalation up to double, one breath at a time. Let's take the following example.

observed inhalation (i)	3 seconds
observed exhalation (e)	2 seconds
next 2-3 breaths	slow down first second of e breath to make e last to 3 seconds
once i:e is rhythmic at	slow down first 2 seconds of the next e to make
2:3 seconds	e last 4 seconds
2:4 seconds	i last 3 seconds
3:4 seconds	e last 5 seconds
3:5 seconds	e last 6 seconds

once i:e is rhythmic at	slow down first 2 seconds of the next e to make
3:6 seconds	i last 4 seconds
4:6 seconds	e last 7 seconds
4:7 seconds	e last 8 seconds

You then work on making I:E: 4:8, 5:8, 5:9, 5:10, and so on. You move on to the next stage only if you can comfortably breathe in the said rhythm. It is possible that when you increase the length of I, your E might become shorter at first. In such a case, go back to the previous ratio and pick it up slowly from there.

The scriptures prescribe a ratio of 10:20 for a beginner, and add breath retention to this rhythm. This prescription for a beginner too, is an advance practice for people like you and me who are most likely to practice for 15-20 minutes in a day. We might take breaks too, when we don't have the time or don't feel like doing the practice. This is normal. Therefore, once your breath ratio begins to effortlessly reach 10:20, I would recommend approaching a trusted and reputed teacher of your choice, who can guide you further on your journey.

BREATHING UNDER STRESS

Once you get into the pattern of observing your breath, you will be capable of noticing the changes in it when under stress. Gradually, you will be able to regulate your breath even as you face a stressful situation. Do we not, after all, ease ourselves with a few sighs, which are nothing but complete exhalations through the mouth when we feel overburdened. Sighing helps to break the cycle of tension. Similarly, a 1-2 minute breather with long, full and smooth exhalations can work wonders.

At such times we must take a moment to adjust the pattern: breathe in and out without straining. At first, the breathing is likely to be erratic. Just observe. Gradually, because we are paying attention to it, the breathing will slow down and start falling into a rhythm. Our agitated thoughts, too, will begin to calm slowly but surely. The best way to defuse anger quickly or decrease frustration is to break the circle of thoughts and take a few conscious breaths. Let the PNS take over for a bit. Breathing with awareness will quieten our emotions and enable us to access our circumstances in a better way.

Let us use an analogy to visualise the process. A movie is made from putting together multiple frames, say 24 frames in a second. If we want to make any changes to the film, it has to be run at a slow speed so that each frame can be seen separately. The frame with the error is then identified and corrected. Similarly, our racing thoughts are like a movie reel that needs to slow down for us to take a look at as we break down the thought process. By exhaling slowly, we can begin to decipher the strain or stress. Our breathing becomes a good barometer for relaxation or stress.

It is important to note that at first, you might find it challenging and overwhelming. It is a slow process, indeed. Persistence, however, pays and success will be ours eventually.

This understanding of conscious breathing is fundamental to all breathing techniques that we will get to in the next chapter. The one takeaway from this section of the book is that you begin with the correct posture and make sure you breathe correctly. The length of your breath will take time to build up, do not worry about that too much.

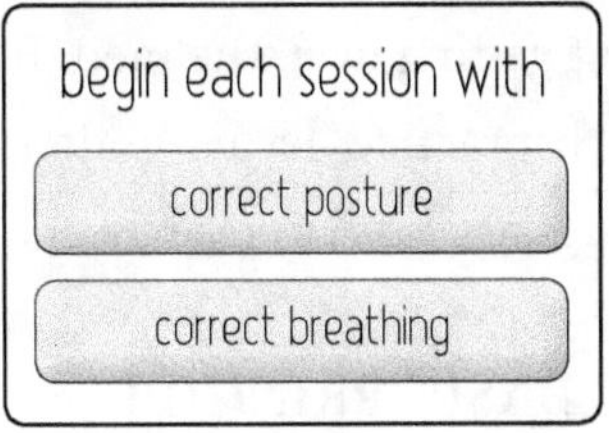

FIVE

THE POWER OF PRANAYAMA

Once we have a decent control over our breathing, we can add pranayama practices to our sessions. We have focussed on practices that are easy to understand and can be performed without any adverse effects. Our aim is to make this practice sustainable over the long term without getting overwhelmed. Before we get into the details of each practice, let us understand some basic principles and language used in pranayama.

BASIC PRINCIPLES

Understand before doing.

The word pranayama is made up of two words—'*prana*' and '*ayama*'. They are understood as 'breath' and 'control', or control over the movement of breath. '*Ayama*' means the action or the voluntary effort to control, direct and regulate this *prana*.

Therefore, pranayama is consciously slowing down and controlling the process of breathing to break the automatic process. This happens as we gain control over breathing by overriding the involuntary control with conscious control. This makes the very fundamental aims of our pranayama practice:

- Taking complete breaths
- Slowing down the breathing rate
- Exhaling more completely and effectively; elongating the exhalations
- Balancing the breaths between the two nostrils
- Building awareness
- Effortless retention of breaths

LANGUAGE OF PRANAYAMA

The above aims can be broken down systematically by thinking of each complete breath as having three processes. The scriptures describe them as *rechaka*, *pooraka*, and *kumbhaka*.

RECHAKA (EXHALATION)

Rechaka is the phase of breathing out smoothly and continuously. In normal breathing, muscular energy is used for inhaling, while exhaling involves merely relaxing the tensed muscles. In pranayamic breathing, the abdominal muscles are under constant control to make the exhalation longer than the inhalation.

Anatomically, the abdomen that may have bulged out during inhalation is contracted and pulled inward with gentle control. This helps evacuate the lungs by raising the diaphragm. The chest contracts and air flows out through the nostrils.

It is crucial to start your conscious breathing practice with the *rechaka*. Unless we first breathe out fully, it is impossible to breathe in correctly.

POORAKA (INHALATION)

Pooraka is the process of drawing in the air smoothly and continuously. After emptying the lungs, the next step is to fill them up to the maximum possible.

Anatomically, when you breathe in deeply, the chest expands, and the diaphragm gets pushed down. The organs inside the abdominal cavity get pushed down, and the front wall of the abdomen gets pushed out.

The process of *pooraka* is theoretically slightly different. The lungs fill up and the diaphragm descends, but the muscles of the front wall of the abdomen and those in the perianal region are kept under constant control, and the abdominal wall gets pushed out, but not completely.

However, if we get unduly stressed trying to keep the abdominal wall in place, we miss the subtler effects on the mind. Therefore, it is essential to breathe as gently as possible with a constant flow and rhythm. We must learn to be aware of the breath inhaled through the nostrils, the flowing air touching the back of the throat and further inside behind the chest bone, the ribs and the chest wall expanding, and the gradual rise in pressure inside the abdominal cavity.

KUMBHAKA, RETENTION

Traditionally, the systematic holding of the breath is called *kumbhaka*. *Kumbhaka* means a pitcher or a pot to hold or retain matter, and in the context of pranayama, it means 'to hold the breath or the movement of air'. As mentioned earlier, *kumbhaka* is such an important part of pranayama that some scriptures use the word *kumbhaka* instead of pranayama.

Breath retention can be categorised in a few ways, which we describe later, but it is vital to proceed with caution. Any breath retention increases the pressure inside the chest cavity and the abdomen. Your body has to be able to deal with the increased pressure without adverse effects.

The traditional techniques available to prolong the pauses between breaths safely are called *bandhas* or locks. They have to be learnt under the able guidance of a trained master and will not be dealt with in this book. Here is a quick theoretical glance at the concept of breath retention. While the time-based *kumbhakas* need guidance, the *kewal kumbhaka* is accessible to us, even as beginners, with the help of the practices outlined further ahead.

TIME-BASED *KUMBHAKA*

Antara kumbhaka or internal retention is when the breath is held after inhaling.

Bahya kumbhaka or external retention is when the breath is held after an exhalation.

MECHANISM-BASED *KUMBHAKA*

Sahita Kumbhaka, Deliberate Breath Retention

Sahita kumbhaka is when either the *bahya* or *antara kumbhaka* is deliberately held. Conscious effort is involved in *sahita kumbhaka*. The bandhas mentioned above come into action here.

When we begin with pranayama practices, we must not hold our breath forcefully but instead breathe naturally and smoothly. Only after a considerable time, when we have mastered the basic breathing exercises and have no contraindications, can we proceed with voluntary breath-holding, *sahita kumbhaka* and that too, under the guidance of a teacher. One is eligible for voluntary breath-holding if one can double the duration of exhalation for a long time with ease and comfort.

Breath retention exercises must be done when we reach the stage where we have improved our ability to breathe in and out, and the exercises do not disturb the breathing-in and breathing-out pattern. Only when we have emptied ourselves of air can we take a new breath, and only when we breath in, can we hold it. So, if we do not breathe out fully, we cannot hold our breath.

The eligibility criterion for *sahita kumbhaka* is one's ability to maintain with ease a ratio of 10:20 seconds between inhalation and exhalation.

Kewal Kumbhaka, Automatic Breath Retention

Kewal kumbhaka is when, in the course of practice, the pause persists without effort or discomfort, unconditioned by place, time and number. This is considered the absolute and pure pause and the fruit of one's pranayama practice.

This is a spontaneous and comfortable cessation of breath for some time. The breathing cycle comes to a standstill automatically while the mind is fully conscious and aware. This state is also known as the 'perfectly peaceful pause' or one of complete rest. Feelings such as urgency, desire, anxiety, fear, hatred, anger, and even hunger and thirst tend to reduce and even disappear when we are in this state.

Physiologically, it allows a better and complete exchange

of gases in the lungs. This leads to a positive impact on all the functions of the body. The metabolic processes in the body decrease in intensity, and the body's oxygen consumption reduces to some extent. We also influence the PNS, lowering the heart rate and blood pressure. This means that when the breath is held effortlessly, our body conserves energy, which can then be used for some other purpose.

Let us quickly recollect what we have read about the correlation between our mental state and our breathing. Agitated thoughts produce rapid, coarse and erratic breathing. At the same time, a calm and composed mind is reflected in slow and smooth breathing. By consciously slowing down the breathing rate, the harmful speed of pointless thoughts comes under control. Ultimately, with the spontaneous cessation of breathing, the mind can experience perfect calm, poise and balance – a near thoughtless state of mind, the optimum condition for health and healing.

This state of utter blissfulness is within reach of one and all. The experience of *kewal kumbhaka* is addictive in a good way—physically, mentally, emotionally and spiritually. If practised regularly, this exercise is more satisfying than a cup of coffee or a cigarette. Almost all of the practices below will make the safe experience of *kewal kumbhaka* accessible to you. Some more than others, as we will point out when applicable.

There are other ways in which a regular practitioner begins to experience *kewal kumbhaka*.

Deliberately slowing down breathing: Rishi Patanjali defines this in the *Patanjali Yoga Sutra* (PYS) as,

Tasmin sati shwasa – praswasha-yorgati-vicchedah pranayamah.

– PYS 2:49

Translated, pranayama means control over the regular pattern of breathing, with a slowing down of the breath (*vicchedah*). This ultimately leads to total and spontaneous silencing of the breath.

Thus, merely slowing down the rate of normal breathing and maintaining its rhythm and smoothness with deeper breaths can lead to *kewal kumbhaka*.

Prolonged and regular practice of *sahita kumbhaka*: The yoga sutra says,

Bahya abyantara-stambha-vrittir-dishakala sankhyabhih paridrishto divgha sukshmah.

– PYS 2.50

This translates to, "The breathing movement can come to a standstill in three ways: *bahya*, after exhaling; *abhyantara*, after inhaling; and *stambha*, either way in between—when the breath stops spontaneously after a long-term practice of the earlier two types."

The *Hatha Yoga Pradipika* (*HYP*), another yogic text, believes that one has to practise many rounds of *sahita kumbhaka* daily over a long period and maintain the *kumbhaka* state for an increasing number of seconds. This will progressively require less physical effort until the stage of *kewal kumbhaka* is reached.

PRANAYAMA VS DEEP-BREATHING

Many regard pranayama as deep-breathing, but fundamentally the two are different.

	Pranayama	*Deep Breathing*
When	One is relaxed and sits intentionally to practise pranayama	Happens secondary to muscular exercise or is done consciously to overcome fatigue
Attitude	With awareness	More mechanical
Aim	Balancing the functions of the autonomic nervous system	Providing more oxygen and ridding the body of accumulated carbon-dioxide
ANS	Towards PNS	Towards SNS. Moves toward PNS after exercise

	Pranayama	*Deep Breathing*
Breathing rate	Slow, aims at slowing down more and more with practice	Fast, when secondary to exercise. Moderate, during conscious breathing
Importance to prolonged exhalation	Yes	No
Heart rate and BP	Slow to begin with and stays that way	High to begin with and reduces with deep breathing
Breath retention	Yes	No
Inhalation-to-exhalation ratio	Followed to make it rhythmic and stay in control	Doesn't need attention

STARTING YOUR PRANAYAMA PRACTICE

Begin the virtuous clean space-calm mind cycle.

Just as a musician prepares for a performance, we, too, have to fine-tune ourselves to set a mood for good practice. Correct posture is indispensable for the successful practice of pranayama.

As physical discomfort and mental chatter are closely interrelated, a stable and calm body that can stay still for the duration of your session is essential. Unnecessary movement dissipates *prana,* so one must be able to sit comfortably in a position for an extended period.

The posture has to be stable (*sthira*) so that minimal effort is required to maintain it. It has to be comfortable (*sukha*) so that your mind is free of distractions. You can adopt any of the postures mentioned in the "Sitting Right, Or Lie Down" section on posture.

CREATING A CONDUCIVE ENVIRONMENT

For healthy progress in pranayama, some preliminary preparation will do us good.

- Practise pranayama in a well-ventilated room. An open-air environment like a balcony, terrace, or garden is even better for beginners. Do not do it in a closed, air-conditioned space where fresh air is restricted.
- If possible, assign a special place for the daily practice.
- Sit on a mat or cushion. Avoid practising sitting on the bare floor.
- Pranayama needs concentration and attention; practise in a distraction-free environment. So, switch off the phones, the TV, the radio, and the call bell to avoid distraction. Or at least minimise such potential interference.
- If possible, bathe with normal tap water before yogic practices. It dispels drowsiness. Avoid bathing for half an hour after you finish pranayama.

- Wear comfortable and loose clothes. If practising outdoors, cover the body with a sheet to avoid disturbance from insects.

- Practise pranayama on an empty stomach, but you should not be feeling hunger pangs either. Wait for at least three hours after a meal. The best time to do pranayama is early morning. Drink a little fruit juice or a small cup of tea or coffee, and wait for thirty minutes or so before starting pranayama.

- Answer the call of nature before you begin your session. If the bowels are constipated, drink warm water on waking up, do asanas like *bhujangasana* (cobra pose), *shalabhasana* (locust pose), and *dhanurasana* (bow pose). With regular practice of asanas and pranayama, you might find relief from your bowel discomforts. If you don't know these poses, do gentle backbends or consult with a knowledgeable teacher.

- You may drink a cup of milk or eat a light snack ten-fifteen minutes after completing pranayama.

- For more significant benefits, avoid smoking and drinking, and if possible, opt for a *satvika* diet.

- Seek a trained yoga teacher, to begin with. So you know your techniques are correct.

- Be regular and systematic with your practice. Missing pranayama will eventually become like missing food.

- Do not practise when you are unwell or have active infections, loose motions, etc.

LISTEN TO YOUR BODY:

UNDER-DO RATHER THAN OVERDO

We have been trained to push ourselves beyond our limits. In pranayama specifically, by pushing too hard, we harm ourselves more than we benefit. Any exaggeration or performance of pranayama when the body is not fully prepared can cause breathing difficulties and symptoms and signs of discomfort such as nervousness, shortness of breath, unstable blood pressure and palpitations. Eventually, we risk losing interest and giving it up altogether. By proceeding slowly and carefully, we not only make it a pleasurable routine but also benefit from it.

Remember, any tension or discomfort during pranayama is a sign that the body and/or mind is not ready for whatever you are trying to do. If you are gasping for air, something needs to change about your practice. On such occasions, go back to the basics—just breathe consciously for a few minutes. Maybe, that day's practice should be only deep, mindful breaths.

UNDERSTAND YOUR LEVEL OF PRACTICE AT THIS MOMENT

Even as you become a regular practitioner, there will be good days and not-so-good days. There will be sessions where you are wholly focussed, and every practice comes with ease, and there will be times when you just cannot concentrate. It is okay. Just stick to your routine, and you will have more good sessions than not. Let your body and mind space lead you to your day's practice rather than having expectations, to begin with. Keep the following guidelines in mind as you start each session, irrespective of how long you have been practising.

EFFORTLESS PRACTICE

Avoid all strain. If you contort the facial muscles during a practice, it means that you are going beyond your capacity. Again, your breath is your guide. If it feels laboured or out-of-rhythm, you are overdoing it and going against the first guideline.

Don't rush. Practise pranayama with a relaxed mind. After each practice, enjoy and appreciate its beneficial effects, and then move on to the next one.

Too much, too soon is bad. Progress slowly and steadily. Do not be in a hurry to get more benefits by increasing the duration of the practice. You should feel fresh and joyful after pranayama. If you feel tired and exhausted, reduce the duration of your session or check for other reasons for the fatigue. Pranayama and breathing exercises should not be pushed to the extent of weariness and exhaustion.

Stay still. Do not shake the body unnecessarily during practice, as this dissipates energy. The posture should be comfortable, steady and firm. Yet, if you experience pain or discomfort, release the discomfort gently, take a break and re-start once the agitation wears off. Often, just observing the discomfort makes it disappear slowly.

Don't tolerate pain. Your body can distinguish between pain that is good for your body and one that isn't. You have to be aware of sweet pain and stop when it doesn't seem right or feels like it is causing injury. The aim of pranayama is to relax and not to induce pain.

Keep expectations at bay. Like anything else in life, expectations are likely to lead to disappointment. For pranayama, it becomes counter-productive. The benefits will come, you should just continue to practise.

Use common sense. If one kind of practice is not agreeable to your system, change or avoid it after consulting your teacher. This is called *yukti*.

Aim for meaningful practice. Practise with awareness and not mechanically. As we practise more regularly, we might become complacent. It is possible that our attitude towards pranayama may become mechanical. The following thought pattern might develop: 'x' pranayama has to be done 'y' number of times, followed by 'c' pranayama for 'd' minutes, and so on. Intent on completing the protocol for the day, we jump from one to the next without being aware of the effects on the body and the mind. This is the time to catch ourselves and make our practice meaningful again. It is about being conscious, about being aware of what your mind is up to.

SPECIAL GUIDELINES FOR BEGINNERS

Anyone can benefit from pranayama by following some basic rules. As long as we pay attention to the reactions of the body, there is nothing to fear. Problems can arise when we alter our breathing and cannot recognise or attend to an adverse bodily reaction.

- Learn pranayama from a compassionate yoga teacher who will guide you and rectify your practice. Your practice will depend on your age, breathing ability, state of health, etc. Faulty techniques can do more harm than good and have to be individually rectified.
- Be sincere, regular and systematic when practising on your own.

- When we just begin to practise, we might find ourselves struggling to breathe deeply. We might feel an urge to take a quick breath between long, slow breaths. We must be patient with ourselves and give ourselves time.

- If we experience difficulty in breathing out, or if the quality of exhalation is not good, the entire pranayama practice gets adversely affected. Practise conscious breathing as described earlier to overcome this issue.

CONTRAINDICATIONS

While each practice has specific contraindications, people suffering from chronic shortness of breath and conditions like emphysema, bronchitis and asthma should not directly begin pranayama. Practise some asanas to first increase the lungs' volume and free the muscles of the ribs, the back and the diaphragm. These should be done under the guidance of a trained teacher. At the beginning of each session too, make sure that the body is warmed up before the breathing exercises.

COMMON BENEFITS

When you are aware, everything is beautiful.

While each pranayama practice we have included in our protocol has specific benefits, some benefits accrue from all the practices. For the sake of convenience and brevity, we have collected the common advantages under this section. Specific benefits will be discussed along with the technique for each pranayama practice.

PHYSIOLOGICAL EFFECTS OF PRANAYAMA

Pranayama helps the functioning of almost each of the body's systems. Here is a brief overview of these advantages.

Respiratory system: At the heart of pranayama practices lies the concept of using the lungs' maximum capacity. This improves the elasticity of the lungs and their functioning through stronger respiratory muscles and better gas exchange. The respiratory rate also slows down with effective pranayama.

Circulatory system: The efficient movement of the diaphragm facilitates a gentle compression and relaxation of the heart as if it were getting a soothing massage. This lowers the heart rate and promotes the formation of natural collateral blood vessels that help to bypass obstruction in the coronary arteries.

Digestive system: Again, the diaphragmatic movement moves abdominal organs. Therefore, the stomach, the intestines, the liver, and the pancreas contract and relax. This massage-like movement improves their functioning and secretions for better digestion.

Nervous system: At the risk of repetition, the very nature of breathing in pranayama positively influences the nervous system as a whole. It affects the higher functions of the Central Nervous System (CNS), such as perception, planning, execution of tasks, learning and memory. It also increases alertness, along with relaxation, as alpha waves dominate the brain's activity, leading to less nervous irritability. This also results in less neuroticism, decreased mental fatigue, and improved awareness.

Regular practice of pranayama over a long period also leads to better circulation to the spinal nerves, better nerve impulse transmission to create an inner balance or homeostasis.

Endocrine system: Pranayama allows richer blood supply to the hormone-secreting glands, leading to balanced glandular activity and hormonal profile. It also decreases the activity of the adrenocortical gland, the endocrine gland, which discharges the stress hormones. This can be interpreted as an increased ability to resist stress.

PRANAYAMA FOR THE MIND

The movement of energy within us also produces thoughts. Thoughts can be considered the content of our minds. We aim to direct this movement to create thoughts that will benefit us rather than cause suffering.

Through pranayama, that is, by exercising control over the breath, we can control the subtle *prana* inside. This control of *prana* means control of the mind, so control of breath is control of both *prana* and the mind.

The *Yoga Sutras* of Rishi Patanjali say,

Tatah shriyate prakaashanarnam

– PYS 2.52

When we practise pranayama, the veil of lethargy and ignorance gradually draws away from the mind, increasing clarity and mind power. This clarity allows the light of wisdom to shine. This wisdom will enable us to discern between helpful and unhelpful thoughts. This capacity pacifies our thought process, creating a mind that has either reduced stress-inducing thoughts or the calm ability to handle stress.

Stress management: Pranayama is the best method of managing stress as it progressively trains the mind to learn to listen to itself. The external sounds and the incessant demands of day-to-day living suppress access to our rational mind.

Under stress, our ANS, designed by nature to protect us, tends to overreact and balances precariously on the threshold. At this juncture, pranayama works by strengthening our inhibitory response to the stress-handling mechanisms of the body.

Positive change in attitude: Conscious, slow, deep and rhythmic breathing brings about a balanced, tranquil and relaxed state of well-being. Our instincts, desires, and ego come under control and cannot interfere with the mind. This brings about a positive behaviour change.

Sharp awareness: Pranayama focuses on bringing the inhalation and the exhalation into a particular relationship with each other. The very act of focusing on these aspects of breathing keeps us alert and aware of what is going on in the mind. This helps draw the mind away from the unhealthy chatter of thoughts.

Third-person attitude: Regular practice helps us control our emotions, resulting in inner calm, balance and *sakshi bhaava*–a third-person attitude, where you experience activities and events in your life as a witness. This brings distance and much-needed perspective and clarity of mind. What psychologists call our rational mind, Indian philosophy calls the witnessing self, which can analyse without getting emotionally carried away.

A still mind: This is the main aim of pranayama. When the mind is at a standstill, no thoughts or emotions disturb it. We can control our temperament, desires, mood swings, and instincts with the practice of pranayama.

Hatha Yoga Pradipika puts this very aptly:

Chale vate chalam chittam, nischale nischalam bhavet, yogi sthanutvamaprotitato vayum nirodhayet

– HYP 2.2

That is, 'As long as breathing continues on its own, the mind remains unstable; when the breath is controlled, the activity of the mind is also controlled.'

Preparation for meditation: With the consistent and committed practice of pranayama, spontaneous pauses start to occur during the phases of breathing. The mind turns absolutely blank, a rare state of stillness and peace for which we all yearn. This happens because the inner chatter of irrational thoughts that keep bombarding our mental frame gets filtered out, and the mind becomes steady, peaceful and more suitable for concentration and meditation.

A PRACTICAL ROUTINE

Regular and sustained steps makes the race fruitful.

Once we have corrected our erroneous breathing patterns, if any, we are ready to embark on our journey to manipulating our breath to control and improve our mental and physical bodies. Here are the practices and routine that I would recommend for a beginner. A lot of the following will sound like mere words. Don't you worry, we will break down the practices in further detail soon. Think of this as a cheat sheet till you become familiar with the techniques and routine.

A Practical Routine

1. posture	• sit with correct and comfortable spine alignment
2. observe breath	• observe current breath flow without control
3. correct errors if any	• reverse to correct • shallow to deep • rapid to slow • erratic to rhythmic • restricted to free-flowing
4. prayer	• any prayer of your choice • aloud or a mental chant
5. gentle exercises	• side-bends and twists • few asanas/rounds of surya namaskara
6. cleansing practices	either of the following or both depending on the level of your practices: • kapalabhati: 3-5 minutes • bhastrika: 20-30 strokes, 3 sets
7. breathing practices	either of the following or both depending on the level of your practices: • anuloma viloma/nadi shuddhi: 5-7 minutes • ujjayi: 5-7 minutes
8. special practices as necessary	• anti-anxiety • anti-depression
9. chanting practices	5-7 minutes of one of the two practices. of course, you can do both • bhramari • om chanting
10. sit in silence	• as long as you can

We will take up each of these in order. We have discussed steps number 1 (posture), 2 (observe breath), and 3 (correct errors, if any) at great length in the previous section. We now move on to the next steps.

Step 4: Prayer

This prayer is not meant to be religious. Step 2 and the prayer in step 4 intend to withdraw your mind from the outer world to the world within. Therefore, this prayer can be a prayer of gratitude and/or commitment to your practice.

Step 5: Gentle stretches or warm-ups

These physical exercises should include spine movements to allow free flow of breath and *prana* in your body. The intention is also to expand your lungs along the length, width and front and back. This extension in all three dimensions will allow fuller breaths. Such stretches also reduce the tightness of underused muscles and prepare your body to sit for a longer time.

The exercises could include anything you like. Allow your body to guide you through these. If you have more time, you could also include some asana practice or a few rounds of surya namaskara, or take a walk before your pranayama session. Some physical exercise is recommended to dispel lethargy and/or stiffness.

It is okay to practice pranayama once in a while without

initial physical exercise. Let lack of time for preliminary exercises not become a reason to skip pranayama. However, physical activity before pranayama sessions is highly recommended.

Please note that these suggestions are for a pranayama session. Your fitness regime will include more intense exercise or asana practice as per your body, personality, likes, comfort and health.

We can now get to the actual breathing practices.

PRANAYAMA PRACTICES

Cleanse. Receive. Organise.

The order in which we proceed is essential because real progress cannot take place haphazardly. When we decide to change the furniture in a room, we proceed by first removing the old items, getting the new ones in and then arranging them properly in the room—cleansing, receiving and organising. Similarly, our pranayama protocol should first cleanse the body and the mind. We then make room to receive and distribute *prana* evenly.

Do keep in mind that after each of these practices take your time to appreciate the after-effects. Many of these practices have a meditative effect. It would not be wise to get out of that state suddenly. Therefore, after each practice:

- Sit in silence for a bit.

- Do not open your eyes suddenly.
- Instead,
    - rub your palms,
    - massage the bones around your eyes,
    - cup your eyes,
    - slowly blink open your eyes behind your palms,
    - increase the distance between your fingers, letting light in,
    - release the palms.

Step 6: Cleansing practices

Kapalabhati and *bhastrika* are breathing techniques used primarily for cleansing our internal organs. They help cleanse the air passage of undesired mucous, the chest of a sensation of tightness, the lungs of carbon dioxide, and the mind of a sense of heaviness and blockage.

Owing to their cleansing properties, *kapalabhati* and *bhastrika* are called *kriya* in yogic terminology, which are to be done before any pranayama. However, since they are breathing practices, some schools of thought refer to them as pranayama, especially *bhastrika*. The duration of *kewal kumbhaka* decides whether the practice is acting as a *kriya* or pranayama. If it is sufficiently long—thirty seconds to one minute—then it is pranayama.

Generally, *kriyas* are prescribed only if you have symptoms that require you to do them. Most ancient scriptures describe 6-8 such cleansing practices. Some of them are quite advanced. Others are so powerful that they shouldn't be done daily. However, considering our exposure to pollution, postural and eating habits, *kapalabhati* and *bhastrika* operate to clean those organs of our body that can do with daily cleaning. Therefore, it is safe to practice them daily in a moderate number of repetitions.

BENEFITS OF *KAPALABHATI* AND *BHASTRIKA*

CLEANSING THE BODY

Our day-to-day breathing habits and hunched or over-arched posture promote the accumulation of toxic gas in the lungs, especially in the lower lobes. Both these cleansing practices promote active and forceful exhalations, primarily encouraging better expulsion of carbon dioxide from the lungs.

BETTER GAS EXCHANGE

While these practices are primarily used to wash out carbon dioxide from the system, in the process, there is an excess supply of oxygen too. Since large quantities of carbon dioxide get washed out, the respiratory centre does not stimulate breathing. This delays the triggering of the next breath. Brain cells that are sensitive to low oxygen levels in the blood do not initiate the next breath because the blood has an adequate amount of oxygen. This delay gives rise to a peaceful pause. This pause allows for a better exchange of gases in the lungs.

CLEANSING THE MIND

The pause mentioned above is *kewal kumbhaka* which we discussed earlier—the fruit of pranayama. In this state, the mind is calm and balanced. While the *kewal kumbhaka* can be experienced after any pranayama practice, it comes easier, quicker, and longer after *kapalabhati* and *bhastrika*. Just a few minutes of the exercise can lead to a longer-than-normal pause and without discomfort. In fact, 10-15 *bhastrika* breaths can sometimes lead to 10-15-second long pauses, if not longer. This cleansing of the mind sets the stage for other pranayama practices and meditation.

INSTANT PEACE OF MIND

Though it is not the aim of these practices, you are likely to experience instant peace of mind after performing either of the two techniques. The pause that follows these practices automatically translates to reduced mental chatter.

We all go through patches in life when we are indecisive, agitated, or disturbed. *Kapalabhati* can be practised for a few minutes as an emergency tool to calm a disturbed state of mind. This rest rejuvenates the mind and clears our minds to lead us to balanced answers to our problems.

KAPALABHATI (Skull-illuminating breath)

Kapalabhati translates to 'that which shines or brings a *bhati* or glow to the *kapala*, forehead. In Sanskrit, *kapala* means skull or forehead, and *bhati* means luminosity and perception. *Kapalabhati* is the practice that brings a state of luminosity or clarity in mind as well as the body.

Kapalabhati breaths involve quick, short, forced exhalations using the abdominal muscles. Inhalations are automatic and diaphragmatic. You can think of it as active exhalations and passive inhalations. In contrast, usually, when we breathe, inhalations are active while exhalations are passive.

The quick and sharp exhalations use the abdominal muscles, while the chest is more or less quiet and relatively motion-free. The abdominal muscles are made to contract actively and with a forceful upward movement. The following automatic inhalation allows the diaphragm to descend easily, reducing the pressure inside the lungs slightly, and the atmospheric air rushes in.

PRECAUTIONS

Over and above the general precautions and preparation necessary for all pranayama practice listed in an earlier section:

- Do not contort the face or squeeze the nostrils. A smile on the face and a calm demeanour will make the practice easy and pleasurable.
- Do not lift the shoulders with each breath.
- Keep the chest expanded and immobile as the breathing is due to active abdominal muscles at work.
- Women should avoid doing this exercise during menstruation or pregnancy.
- *Kapalabhati* should not be practised by anyone suffering from uncontrolled or severe hypertension, active heart disease, vertigo, glaucoma, a bleeding nose, fluid in the ears, epilepsy, hernia, reflux oesophagitis, a gastric ulcer, or a slipped disc.
- Avoid *kapalabhati* if you are suffering from
  i) congested ears or nose,
  ii) a bad stomach.

TECHNIQUE

- It is assumed that you have performed steps 1 to 5 of the protocol, as it applies to you.
- Make sure you are in a comfortable sitting position with your spine erect while maintaining its natural curve. The position must be such that the belly muscles are relaxed and can move freely and actively, keeping the body steady and comfortable.
- Cup your palms facing down on the thighs or knees,

and very gently press them. This helps lift the spine and pushes the shoulders back.

- Relax the nose and soften the face with a gentle smile.
- Exhale completely.
- Inhale and expand your chest, and maintaining the expanded chest, start the practice.
- Forcefully exhale with your nose using your abdominal muscles. The belly button will be pulled in towards the spine, and up towards the heart as if it were making an inverted L. Effectively, you are pushing air out of the lungs with a strong flapping movement of the abdomen in an upward direction.
- Allow inhalation to happen automatically as the abdominal muscles relax. It is smooth and effortless and prepares you for the next thrust of the abdomen.
- Forcefully exhale again. This would be your second *kapalabhati* stroke.
- As a beginner, do ten-twenty expulsions per round, at the rate of one second for exhalation and two-three seconds for inhalation, resting between the rounds. Do two or three rounds.
- Gradually, over a few weeks, you can move on to about 20-40 strokes in one round.
  - The guideline, as usual, is your breath and body. You shouldn't feel out of breath, nor should you feel pain or discomfort in any part of your body.

- You shouldn't feel fatigued or dizzy either.
- If you experience any of the above, stop the practice for a minute or so and start again. You could consider stopping for the day, too, depending on what your body is telling you. Like with any yogic practice, stay within your capacity. It is not a competitive activity.
- Your speed should be approximately 50-60 strokes per minute.
- At the end of one round, take a short rest. There will be an automatic suspension of breathing. This is *kewal kumbhaka*. The urge to breathe stops for a few seconds. Sit very still and observe the body and mind, and experience the feeling of peace. Enjoy this state of deep rest and freshness. Wait until the breath automatically resumes and then go on to the next round.
- Do three such rounds.

• Exhalations should be regular and consistent, like the ticking of a clock. Jerky and erratic breaths will lead to hunger for air in the form of intermittent gasping for breath. The rhythm should be slow and steady.

• Correct practice of *kapalabhati* produces a crisp sound as one exhales without any facial contortions. The sound is produced by the volume of air being pushed up by the forceful action of the diaphragm, not the muscles of the chest, the shoulders, the neck or the face. Yet, the sound is not very loud. A person sitting next to you shouldn't even realise that you are breathing any different. If you find yourself producing loud noises,

- relax your facial muscles, smile from within, and
- pay attention to the movement of your abdomen.
- Inhalations are silent.
- As you progress in your practice, over months, you can increase the number of strokes per round to
  - three rounds of 50-70
  - two rounds of 75
  - one round of 150
  - two rounds of 100
  - one round of 200, and so on.
  - Do not go over 300 strokes.
- As you progress, over months or even years, you can also increase your speed to 100-120 strokes per minute. Do not go faster than that. It is essential not to sacrifice the force of the abdominal contraction to achieve a greater speed.
- Be prepared for the fact that you might go two steps ahead and one step behind. Respect your body and mind's language in each individual session.

Modified Technique for Beginners

If you are not able to get the technique right. Try one of the following.

Push palm in: Place one palm on your belly. Every time you exhale, allow your palm to gently push the belly in and up. Allow the belly to relax and palm to come outward with the passive inhalation. After a few rounds, you might begin to get the technique.

Mouth exhalations: Imagine a lit candle about 8-10 inches away from your mouth. For every exhalation, blow out through your mouth to extinguish the flame. You will observe the belly automatically following the required pattern. Once you get the rhythm, try to blow out the imaginary candle through your nose exhalations.

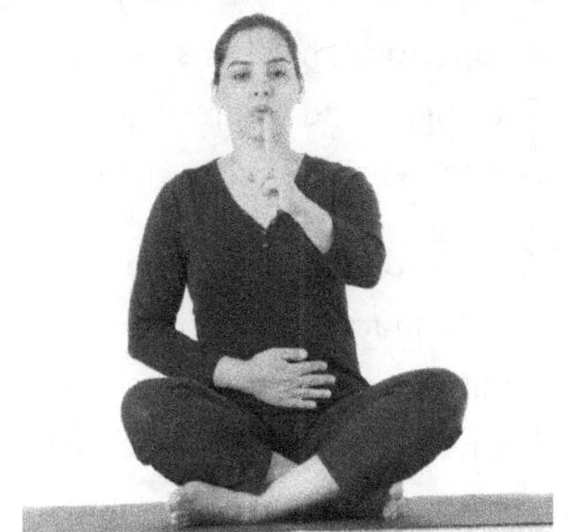

kapalabhati-blowing technique for beginners

COMMON OBSERVATIONS

The belly protrudes during active exhalation: This means that you are unknowingly a reverse breather. You must first correct this; follow the technique explained in the earlier section on 'Conscious Breathing'. If you are not a reverse breather, try "pushing palm in" and/or the "mouth exhalations" techniques mentioned above to correct the pattern.

Pressure in the perineum area or lower body: This would mean your muscular activity is aiming downward towards the lower body rather than upward towards the chest cavity. You can correct this habit by retraining the abdominal muscles to contract upward during normal exhalations, like when you cough or sneeze. If left uncorrected, it can lead to problems like incontinence.

No pause after each round: It is likely that you are not giving enough time for inhalations between your active exhalations. You might find yourself gasping for breath. Reduce the speed, thereby allowing passive in-breaths.

Mind jumps from thought to thought: You might have become so used to the practice that it has become mechanical. You can remedy this by gently bringing your mind back to the abdominal movement whenever you catch it wandering away from the practice. You can also count your strokes to keep your mind focused on your practice.

BENEFITS

In addition to the common benefits accrued from pranayama and other cleansing breaths, *kapalabhati*:

- Cleans the nasal passageway and the sinuses.
- Cleans the respiratory tract and alleviates mucous disorders.
- Expels the stagnant air in the lower lobes of the lungs, which remains there due to shallow breathing and undesirable sitting postures.
- Increases lung capacity, benefiting people suffering from respiratory disorders. The volume of air taken in during this breathing is only 150-200 ml per breath. However, the total air taken per minute is more than usual due to the higher breathing rate.
- Clears the mind when you are feeling heavy or foggy in the head.
- Strengthens and makes the abdominal muscles flexible.
- Alleviates digestive problems like constipation.
- Relieves backache, which is caused not just by weak muscles but also by the weak abdominal wall compounded with a protruding belly. A distended abdomen pulls the back forward, distorting the spinal alignment and stretching the back muscles, resulting in a spasm. *Kapalabhati* helps relieve backache

by strengthening the muscles of the back and the abdomen.

- Improves posture.
- Dispels lethargy and drowsiness.
- Brings a glow to the face.

Other physiological effects during and after the practice are as follows:

- The heart rate increases slightly by fifteen-twenty beats per minute. But, the pause restores and even reduces the heart rate. Continued practice over a long term will also result in a healthy heart rate.
- The systolic blood pressure increases by 7-10 mm Hg. This is why people suffering from uncontrolled high blood pressure should not do this practice. The diastolic blood pressure, however, remains more or less the same.
- There is a slight increase in the sympathetic tone in the body, followed by a parasympathetic predominance after the practice. The result is a balance between the sympathetic and the parasympathetic and brings about a feeling of relaxation.

BHASTRIKA (Bellow breath)

'*Bhastrika*' means bellows, a blacksmith's device to blow air into a fire while working on iron. It is a contraption with an airbag that emits a stream of air when squeezed together with two handles.

Bhastrika consists basically of forced, rapid, deep breathing. We use our chest as bellows. Both inhalations and exhalations are active, sharp and forceful. However, the emphasis is greater on the expulsion of air.

Bhastrika is thoracic chest-breathing, unlike *kapalabhati*.

It is recommended that you learn *bhastrika* under a trained teacher before practising on your own.

PRECAUTIONS

If you feel giddy or light-headed, reduce the number of breaths per round or practise a modified, safer version described below.

TECHNIQUE

- It is assumed that you have performed steps 1 to 5 of the protocol, as it applies to you.
- You can perform *bhastrika* by itself or after *kapalabhati*, depending on your level of practice.
- Make sure you are in a comfortable sitting position with your spine erect while maintaining its natural curve. The position must be such that the belly muscles are relaxed and can move freely and actively, keeping the body steady and comfortable.
- Relax the body and mind with a gentle smile.

- Exhale completely.
- As you take a sharp and short inhalation with your nose, expand your chest.
- As you exhale through your nose, the chest contracts and returns to its normal position.
- As a beginner, keep your breath rate slow.
  - Start with 5-10 breaths.
  - You can gradually increase to 30-40 breaths per round. To go beyond this count, you should consult a trained teacher.
  - It is more important to breathe completely with concentration rather than aim for a faster rate.
- After the final expulsion, inhale slowly and deeply.
- Then slowly exhale as deeply as possible.
- At this point, the breath stops on its own. Enjoy the pause and the calmness that it brings.
- When your breath returns to normal, you have completed one round of *bhastrika*.
- Rest for a bit, taking a few normal breaths.
- Do 2-3 rounds.

Modified Technique for Beginners

The body takes time to adjust to the rapid alterations in carbon dioxide levels. As a beginner, it is normal to experience light-headedness or giddiness. A simpler version is to practise active breathing with shoulder-shrugging.

- Sit comfortably with the spine erect and place your palms on your thighs or knees.
- With every inhalation, raise your shoulders towards the ears.
- With every exhalation, lower your shoulders.
- The rhythm of the breath is coordinated with the rhythm of the shoulder shrugs.

BENEFITS

Overall, the precautions and the benefits of *bhastrika* are the same as *kapalabhati*. Some specific benefits of *bhastrika* are:

- Relieves throat inflammation.
- Increases gastric fire and improves digestion.
- Alleviates diseases of the nose and the chest.
- Improves appetite.
- Warms the body.
- Prolongs the *kewal kumbhaka*, improving all benefits derived from *kewal kumbhaka*

Step 7: Breathing practices

We will describe two simple practices. Both can be done by almost anyone. There are hardly any contraindications. In any one session, you can incorporate either practice. However, your session will be more rounded and complete if you practise both.

ANULOMA VILOMA OR *NADI SHUDDHI* (Alternate Nostril Breathing)

Yogic texts use various terms for this practice—*anuloma viloma, nadi shodhanam, nadi shuddhi* and *sukha purvaka pranayama*. We can translate it to alternate nostril breathing.

The practice consists of slow, deep, quiet breathing, using one nostril at a time. Each breath is as slow and as comfortable, using full lung capacity, as it is in the complete breath. The right thumb and the ring finger are used to close the right and left nostrils, respectively. Left-handers can use their left thumb and left ring finger to close the left and right nostrils, respectively.

We know from an earlier discussion that our normal breathing dominates alternately between the two nostrils at different times during the day. In a healthy person, this alternation of breath occurs roughly every one-and-a-half to two hours. However, this normal rhythm gets disturbed in most of us and varies considerably, leading to reduced vitality and ill health.

To make the pattern and flow of breath more natural and healthier, we need to regulate and balance our breath. *Nadi shuddhi* was developed to rebalance the equilibrium of breathing. Through this balancing, this practice brings about symmetry between the SNS and the PNS.

There are three variations described in the texts depending on the pattern you follow to switch breaths.

- Switch nostril after each inhalation.
- Exhale through one nostril and inhale through the other. After a few cycles, change sides.
- Inhale and exhale through one side. After a few cycles, change side.

We have described the technique for the first variation. The other two would follow the same technique, except the point at which the nostrils are switched.

PRECAUTIONS

Over and above the general preparatory guidelines for all pranayama, pay special attention to the following:

- During the practice, do not bend the head forward
- Do not apply too much pressure on the nostrils such that the nose tilts to one side.
- If you find your mind wavering too much with thoughts in any session, stop the practice and skip to chanting.

TECHNIQUE

- Irrespective of the nostril you are breathing through, you will practise 'conscious breathing'.
- All basic 'conscious breathing' fundamentals apply.
- Sit comfortably in any posture with ease.
- Relax the facial muscles with a gentle smile.

- All the directions below are for right-handed people. Left-handed people can use their left hand and follow the steps in mirror image.
- With the right hand, make a gentle fist and release the thumb and the ring finger. This hand position is called the *nasika mudra*. If this position is uncomfortable, you can use the thumb and the index finger.
- Gently close your right nostril with your right thumb and exhale completely through the left nostril.
- Inhale slowly and deeply through your left nostril.
- Gently close the left nostril with the right ring finger and release the right nostril.
- Exhale slowly and completely through the right nostril.
- Inhale deeply through the same (right) nostril.
- Gently close the right nostril with your right thumb and release the left nostril.
- Exhale through the left nostril.
- This completes one cycle of *anuloma viloma* or *nadi shuddhi*. Therefore, two complete breaths make one cycle.
- Continue this pattern of exhale-inhale-switch-exhale-inhale-switch, switching from one nostril to the other.
- End the practice with a left nostril exhalation.
- Allow the hands to rest on the lap and sit still with eyes closed. Observe the stillness in breath and mind.

- After getting comfortable with the pattern of alternate-nostril breathing, we can begin to regulate the timing and bring balance to both nostrils.
- Like with conscious breathing, initially, establish a 1:1 ratio between the inhalations and the exhalations.
- Begin by counting mentally or timing the duration with the ticking of a wall clock. Each person's breath will differ in length.
- Continue to increase the duration. It may vary each day. It is advisable to begin each day afresh. Do not attempt to start from where you left off the previous day. Be slow and gentle in expanding the count. Instead of setting up a scenario for failure, set up one for comfort and ease, and you might find that the closed nostril automatically opens.
- When you are comfortable with a count for five full cycles, increase the length of the exhalations. Start with 4:5, then go on to 4:6 and so on, till the exhalation is twice as long as the inhalation. You can then progress like we did with conscious breathing.
- Savour the breath by letting it out more slowly. Starting the exhalation with a blast produces stress. We are exhausted by the blast and cannot increase the duration of the exhalation. On the other hand, if we start slowly, we can slow down the breath let out in the first two seconds of the breath to slow down the

entire exhalation. As we gain control, it takes longer to breathe out completely.

- With time, practice and patience, it will be possible to attain ratios of 5:10 or 6:12, and even 7:14, 8:16 and 10:20.
- The test of progress is the comfort you feel at the end of practice. With ratios of 5:10, we take just four breaths per minute, and there is no breathlessness, dizziness or discomfort. The body learns to economise and utilise the exchange better, and the mind, too, feels more in tune with the process.
- If you recall our discussion on single nostril breathing, you will not be surprised if the breath length is different through the different nostrils. As you practice, this rhythm will settle in. If for some reason, a pattern is elusive, work with lower ratios. Remember, we are not aiming to achieve targets. We want the best practice possible for the current session, to the best of our present capacity.

THREE LEVELS

- Beginners should attempt to make the duration of inhalation and exhalation equal and do only about six cycles of breathing.
- With practice, the duration of exhalation is slowly

extended to twice the duration of inhalation, and the practice is continued for several minutes.

- Advanced practitioners continue for ten to twenty minutes or longer. They also include voluntary breath retention after inhalation and/or exhalation. One is eligible to attempt this voluntary breath-holding only after
    - reaching a 10:20 second inhalation:exhalation ratio
    - with comfort and ease
    - for many rounds

It is recommended to continue this advanced practice with guidance from an experienced teacher.

BENEFITS

Over and above the common benefits, *anuloma viloma*
- Unblocks and thus balances the flow of vital energy, *prana*, between the two arms of the nervous system. This, in turn, brings an overall sense of balance to the mind and body.
- Longer exhalations allow the PNS to get the upper hand over the SNS. This helps break the vicious cycle of stress and disease. We give more time to the healing mechanisms in the body to take over, thus alleviating our physical and emotional problems.
- Reduces elevated blood pressure, acidity and other effects of high stress.

UJJAYI (Breath of victory)

Ujjayi means 'the victorious one' in Sanskrit or the one that helps gain victory over oneself.

Ujjayi consists of very slow breaths, at about 3-4 breaths per minute. Airflow is restricted by keeping the voice box area in the throat partially closed. The air rubs across the surfaces to produce a soft, uniform, low hissing sound. The mind is focused on breathing, particularly on the low hissing sound.

TECHNIQUE

- All basic 'conscious breathing' fundamentals apply.
- Sit comfortably in any posture with ease.
- Relax the facial muscles with a gentle smile. This will not only relax you but also prevent you from overdoing the practice to a strenuous degree.
- Bring your awareness to your throat. Visualise a tiny hole at the front of your throat. Imagine you are breathing in and out through this hole. This way, you partially tighten the larynx, and the air passes slowly through the throat, producing the hissing sound.
- The sound should have a low and uniform pitch and should be pleasant to hear. It should not be audible to people around you.
- As a beginner, it is possible that you find either inhaling or exhaling with *ujjayi* is more accessible

than the other. If this is the case, use *ujjayi* for the one that feels easier. You can gradually, over weeks of practice, add *ujjayi* for the other part too.

- Hatha Yoga texts emphasise exhalation through the left nostril. But, it is okay to exhale through both nostrils too.
- As we know by now, the length of the exhalation should be about twice that of the inhalation.
- Either way, after completely exhaling through the left or both nostrils, the breath stops automatically before inhalation. Relax and enjoy this *kewal kumbhaka* as long as it is comfortably possible.
- This constitutes one round of *ujjayi*.
- A minimum of nine rounds is recommended.
- Advanced practitioners can include breath retention after inhalation or after exhalation. This should be done under the guidance of a capable teacher.
- *Ujjayi* breaths can also be coordinated with the mental chant of a mantra such as 'So Hum' or 'Om Om'. 'So' during inhalation and 'Hum' during exhalation, or one 'Om' each with inhalation and exhalation.

BENEFITS

Over and above the general benefits of all pranayama, *ujjayi*:

- Strengthens the epiglottis muscles, thus reducing snoring.

- Improves the voice, helps it to become melodious, and enables pitch modulation.
- Relieves tonsillitis, colds and sore throat, asthma, excessive hiccups and a hypersensitive throat.
- Reduces anxiety.
- Improves awareness.
- It is the only pranayama that can be done standing, while walking, or lying down.
- When done with chanting, the hissing sound guides the mental chant, producing an even more balanced state of mind.
- Guides you towards meditation.

For further assistance in following these instructions, visit https://www.youtube.com/watch?v=1DPc85dGh1o or scan the QR code for a free video showing these techniques.

Step 8: Special practices as necessary

Experiencing stress and pain is unavoidable. It is a part and parcel of life, in which you love and care for people, have ambitions for yourself and take risks accordingly. Many a time, the stress doesn't come from an actual stressful event but it is triggered by reliving a past event or by anticipating an undesirable one. In either case, the effect on the body and mind is almost the same as actually going through the situation.

Almost all of us find something or the other to worry about. As a part of our daily life many of us experience varying psychological stressors such as fear, anxiety, shame, anticipatory worry, and perceived threats. This keeps the stress response engaged constantly. One cannot really avoid stress and stressors. But, we can learn how to manage and cope with it.

Special breathing techniques can be used to build resilience. The function of our breath as a connector between our nervous and endocrinal systems can be used to slowly but surely replace our negative feedback system with a more constructive one.

VILOMA VARIATION (ANTI-DEPRESSION)

SPECIFIC BENEFITS

Of course, the first aim and benefit of this practice is to reduce depressive thoughts over time. The breaking of breathing into parts during inhalation and exhalation also induce a *kewal kumbhaka*, which in turn, contributes to a calm mind.

TECHNIQUE

Part 1: Tic-Toc Hand Movement + Viloma Breathing

- All basic 'conscious breathing' fundamentals apply.
- Sit comfortably in any posture with ease.
- Relax the facial muscles with a gentle smile.
- The entire practice is to be done with nose breathing.
- Practise breaking the inhalation into 8 parts with tiny pauses between two parts. Exhale normally. Practise until you are comfortable.
- Practise breaking the exhalation into 8 parts with tiny pauses between two parts. Inhale normally. Do it until you are comfortable.
- Practise breaking both the inhalations and exhalations into 8 parts with tiny pauses between two parts. Do it until you are comfortable.
- This is one part of the practice.
- Now, bend your arms at the elbows, with upper arms close to the rib cage and forearms parallel to the floor hovering above the legs.
- Turn the right palm so that it faces downward and the left palm faces upward.
- Now, inhale and exhale in eight parts as you practised earlier.
- After your breathing settles into a rhythm, move one

hand down and the other hand up simultaneously with each part of the breath. Alternate the hands in rhythm with the breath parts, one hand moving up as the other moves down. The movement of the hands is slight, approximately 6-8 inches, as if bouncing a ball.

- Continue for 3 minutes.
- Change the hand position so that the left palm faces downward and the right palm faces upward.
- Continue for another 3 minutes.
- Change the hand position again for the last three minutes.
- The total time is 9 minutes.

Part 2: Slow and Deep Breathing

- After 9 minutes of the practice, relax the hands on your lap.
- Close your eyes, internally focus on the centre point of the chin. This requires pulling the eyes downwards.
- Breathe slowly and deeply through the nose.
- Try to quieten the mind and avoid engaging with thoughts.
- The total time for this is 3 minutes.

Part 3: Internal Breath Retention

- For the next three breaths, after each inhalation, hold your breath for about 15 seconds each, or to your capacity, without overwhelming yourself.

- Place your hands in fists in three different positions for each internal retention.
- These three positions are
  - Fists against your chest.
  - Fists beside shoulders, elbows bent.
  - Fists against the navel.
- After each internal retention, exhale forcefully through the mouth and release the fist.

Part 4: Relax

Relax in the lying down position for at least 2-3 minutes.

For further assistance in following these instructions, visit https://youtu.be/mMOqRBMpIs4 or scan the QR code for a free video showing this technique.

SHEETALI VARIATION (ANTI-ANXIETY)

SPECIFIC BENEFITS

Sheetali is a cooling down practice that is prescribed in ancient texts. The mouth inhalations and exhalations lower acidic refluxes in the body. The practice cools down the chatter of an anxious mind.

TECHNIQUE

Part 1: Mudra

- Place one palm over the other.
- Cross the top palm's thumb over the bottom palm's thumb.
- Place the crossed hands towards the chest, facing the chest.
- The palms don't touch the chest.

Part 2: Drishti

- Turn your eyes towards the tip of your nose.
- Try to keep your eyes on the tip of your nose through the practice.
- If your eyes tire, take a break by closing them for some time.

Part 3: Breath cycle

- Each breath cycle is composed of four breaths.
- Each breath is one inhalation and the exhalation that follows.
- The four breaths follow a specific pattern of either nose or mouth inhalation and nose or mouth exhalation.
- Whenever you breathe in or out through your nose, it is normal slow breaths.
- When you breathe in through the mouth, you pout as

if you are whistling and suck in air as if you are doing it through a straw.

- When you breathe out through the mouth, it is like a sigh.
- Breath 1: Inhale through the nose, exhale through the nose.
- Breath 2: Inhale through the mouth, exhale through the mouth.
- Breath 3: Inhale through the nose, exhale through the mouth.
- Breath 4: Inhale through the mouth, exhale through the nose.
- So it is
  - Nose-nose
  - Mouth-mouth
  - Nose-mouth
  - Mouth-nose
  - These four breaths make one round. Do 3-4 rounds.

Part 4: Relax

- Release the mudra, bring your palms on your lap.
- Close your eyes.
- Just be with the after-effects of the practice for as long as you can. The thoughts racing through your mind have reduced, slowed down or maybe are even gone.

For further assistance in following these instructions, visit https://youtu.be/icBM6LxfJqg or scan the QR code for a free video showing this technique.

Step 9: Chanting practices

Resonance is a phenomenon where the matching of frequencies from two sources produces higher amplitude waves as they complement each other. The tuning of a stringed musical instrument is an example of resonance. Proper tuning of the strings produces a beautiful sound.

A similar fine-tuning has to be done to find the chant pitch that resonates best with you. Whether *bhramari* or om, chant five times, each at a different pitch, while observing which sound vibrates the most in the body, particularly the head region. While this sounds abstract, you will experience it when you try it.

When you chant, the tongue interacts with the upper palate, the roof of the mouth. The hard palate has sound-and-vibration sensitive points that get stimulated as the tongue touches them. Anatomically, the hypothalamus lies in close proximity to the palate bone. The resonance gets transmitted through the sensitive points on the palate affecting the regional metabolism of the hypothalamus. Different sounds affect different parts of the hypothalamus.

BHRAMARI PRANAYAMA (Humming bee chant)

The word '*bhramari*' is Sanskrit for a female bee. In *Bhramari* pranayama, a humming sound is generated during a slow exhalation, resembling the sound produced by a female bee. Yogis did this pranayama for long durations to experience an ecstatic state of mind.

PRECAUTIONS

Never over-chant or extend your chant into a squeal. Feeling the relaxing vibrations is more important than the duration of the chant.

Again, if you feel breathless and need to inhale immediately after the chant is over, you are over-chanting. The solution is to under-chant slightly, that is, stop one or two seconds before you feel you will run out of breath.

TECHNIQUE

- Sit comfortably in any posture with ease.
- Relax the facial muscles with a gentle smile.
- Gently press the tips of the index finger and the thumb of each hand together in *chin mudra*. Place the palms facing up on your thighs, closer to the knees, with elbows tucked in towards the body. Alternately, place palms one over the other facing the ceiling, on the lap.

- Lips should be closed, but the rows of teeth should be separated, and the tongue relaxed, just behind the lower set of teeth. One can lightly touch the tip of the tongue to the roof of the mouth in what is known as the *khechari mudra*.
- Take a long and deep breath in.
- As you exhale, make a low-pitched humming sound 'mmm' or 'nnn'.
- Feel the humming sound behind the soft palate and within the head.
- Observe the automatic, even if tiny, pause after your exhalation. During this *kewal kumbhaka*, the vibrations resonate throughout the body even though the humming has stopped.
- This completes one round of *bhramari*.
- In the beginning, 5-10 rounds of *bhramari* are enough. Slowly, the practice can be increased to five or ten minutes.

  Some schools emphasise a mudra, a hand gesture, to internalise the sounds and make the practice more effective. If you would like to try this,
- Place the thumbs on the flaps of the ears, pressing them back.
- Lightly place the index finger on the closed eyelids to keep out any external light.
- Place the middle finger on the sides of the nose, allowing it to remain open.

- Rest the ring finger on the part above your upper lip.
- The little finger lies between your lower lips and chin.
- Point the elbow outward away from the head. However, if your arms start hurting, you will get distracted by the discomfort, and you may miss the vibrations and the resonance generated. In such a case, you can let go of the mudra and adopt any of the earlier mudras described above.

BENEFITS

Over and above the general benefits of all pranayama practices, *bhramari*

- Sensitises the body and body systems to healing.
- Cultivates the voice and improves it by increasing the pitch and the melody.
- Strengthens the throat and tonsils by improving circulation and eliminating throat ailments.
- Has a massaging and balancing effect on the thyroid gland.
- Speeds up the healing of tissues all over the body and is a good practice after any surgery.
- Improves memory and concentration.
- Induces a meditative state.

OM CHANTING

Om is the symbol or the verbal expression of creation. Although om is not given any specific definition, it is considered to be a primordial sound. The syllable 'om' is not specific to Indian culture. It has significance in other religions, too. The word 'amen' used among Christians, too, is said to be derived from the syllable 'om'. It means 'May it be so'. In Arabic, a similar term, 'amin', has religious significance.

Om is also used to signify divinity and authority. In the English language, the syllable 'om' occurs in words such as omniscience, meaning infinite knowledge, omnipotent, meaning one with limitless powers, and omnivorous, meaning eating everything. This syllable also appears in words such as omen, which means a sign of something that is to occur in future, or ombudsman, meaning a person having the authority to pronounce a verdict.

Chanting 'om' generates specific vibrations that have a profound effect on us. After a comfortable deep breath, one can start exhaling with the chant of 'ooo', slowly tapering it into 'mmm', and continuing till one can exhale comfortably. The abdominal wall goes inward gradually as you chant, expelling air from your chest.

The chant should be comfortable so that there is no distress in the form of gasping for air immediately after the chant gets over. Kulvalyanandji, founder of the renown Kaivalyadham Health and Yoga Research Center, Lonavala, India, advised that after the chant, the abdomen should be allowed to relax, accompanied by a slight inhalation. Then, one can experience the pause and the stillness without taking any breath till the desire to take the next breath arises.

The chanting of om can be done in three progressive ways:

- Audible chant
- Soft whisper
- Mental chant

Initially, it is better to chant aloud as it helps erase our inhibitions, which are an obstacle to healing. One can then proceed to a soft whisper, audible only to oneself. Ultimately, as the awareness increases, one moves to a mental chant. If you tend to fall asleep during a mental chant, start reciting it out loud again.

By chanting 'om', the mind gradually becomes tranquil, and all the restlessness, worries and tensions disappear. The desire to continue the mental chant also disappears, and one feels like indulging in a state of silence. This feeling of inner silence emerges without any force to concentrate. Therefore, chanting should be done lovingly in a relaxed manner.

ALTERNATIVE METHOD OF CHANTING

Om is made of three and a half syllables: A, O, and M, followed by silence.

We can chant om by dividing the chant into three equal parts: one-third for 'aaa', one-third for 'ooo' and one-third for 'mmm', blending one with the other. Simultaneously, one can feel the movement of the vibrations from the navel to the chest, the throat, and then to the face and head. After a chant, one experiences silence. Then after an inhalation, one proceeds with the following chant.

Step 10: Sit in silence

End each session with a few breaths or, if possible, minutes of silence. Here you just observe without interfering with the nature of chatter in your mind or quietude. Do not engage with any thought. Just be.

Each pranayama practice session will include steps 1 to 10. The quantity and duration of steps 6-9 will depend on the level of your practice. The following table is a rough guideline. You progress from beginner to intermediate levels of practice very gradually, over weeks, adding a few strokes/breaths/minutes at a time.

Happy practicing!

	Beginner	*Intermediate*
1. Posture	Sit with correct and comfortable spine alignment	
2. Observe breath	Observe current breath flow without control	
3. Correct errors, if any	Reverse to correct Shallow to deep Rapid to slow Erratic to rhythmic Restricted to free-flowing	
4. Prayer	Any prayer of your choice. Aloud or a mental chant.	

	Beginner	Intermediate
5. Gentle exercise	Side-bends, twists and/or Gentle asanas and/or Few rounds of surya namaskara	
6. Cleansing practices	Either of the following or both	
Kapalabhati	3 rounds of 20-40 strokes each	1 round of 300 strokes
Bhastrika	3 rounds of 5-10 breaths each	3 rounds of 25-30 strokes
7. Breathing practices	Either of the following or both	
Anuloma Viloma	5 rounds (10 breaths)	10 minutes
Ujjayi	breaths	10 minutes
8. Special practices	Either of the following or both, depending on your need	
Anti-depression	breaths	10 minutes
Anti-anxiety	3-4 rounds	10 minutes
9. Chanting practices	Either of the following or both	
Bhramari	11 chants	10 minutes
OM chanting	11 chants	10 minutes
10. Sit in silence	As long as you can	

Advanced level practitioners should work under the guidance of a trained teacher.

SIX

OUR HEALTH LIES IN OUR OWN HANDS

Arguably, most of us want to be at a better place in the future than where we are today.

If we are physically unwell, we obviously want to be free of the pain. If we cannot be free of our suffering, we want to manage it in a way that it causes the least discomfort. Our suboptimal physical health could be a cause of imbalance in our mental health.

Caused by physical illness or stemming out of unrelated causes, we could be mentally and emotionally unwell. Again, those of us who suffer want to be liberated from low energy levels, depression, anxiety, mood changes and the like. At the very least, we want more good days than bad.

If we are physically and mentally well, we want to sustain good health.

Whatever the level of our physical, mental and emotional health, we want to use the tools at hand, modern or ancient, to be in a better place—a calmer mind and more peaceful state of being.

Sure, we have modern medicine to bring relief from symptoms as much as possible. The use of ancient techniques like pranayama can go hand-in-hand to improve our health holistically. In fact, regular and sustained practice brings us closer to spiritual growth which empowers us to look beyond our physical and mental strains, even as we suffer from them.

Hopefully, this book allows you to begin this journey. Remember, it is a slow process. Know that each practice session is likely to bring a different experience. Respect the difference and trust the process. Take guidance when necessary. Be consistent.

Here's to tiny changes in our day-to-day lives!

JAICO PUBLISHING HOUSE

Elevate Your Life. Transform Your World.

ESTABLISHED IN 1946, Jaico Publishing House is home to world-transforming authors such as Sri Sri Paramahansa Yogananda, Osho, the Dalai Lama, Sri Sri Ravi Shankar, Sadhguru, Robin Sharma, Deepak Chopra, Jack Canfield, Eknath Easwaran, Devdutt Pattanaik, Khushwant Singh, John Maxwell, Brian Tracy, and Stephen Hawking.

Our late founder Mr. Jaman Shah first established Jaico as a book distribution company. Sensing that independence was around the corner, he aptly named his company Jaico ('Jai' means victory in Hindi). In order to service the significant demand for affordable books in a developing nation, Mr. Shah initiated Jaico's own publications. Jaico was India's first publisher of paperback books in the English language.

While self-help, religion and philosophy, mind/body/spirit, and business titles form the cornerstone of our non-fiction list, we publish an exciting range of travel, current affairs, biography, and popular science books as well. Our renewed focus on popular fiction is evident in our new titles by a host of fresh young talent from India and abroad. Jaico's recently established translations division translates selected English content into nine regional languages.

Jaico distributes its own titles. With its headquarters in Mumbai, Jaico has branches in Ahmedabad, Bangalore, Chennai, Delhi, Hyderabad, and Kolkata.

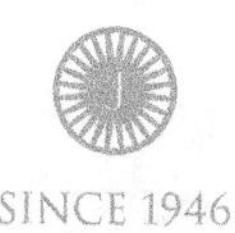

SINCE 1946